IMMUNE
BOOSTERS

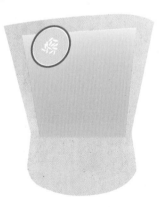

spruce

Safety Note

Immune Boosters should not be considered a replacement for professional medical treatment; a physician should be consulted on all matters relating to health. While the advice and information in this book is believed to be accurate, the publisher cannot accept any legal responsibility or liability for any injury or illness sustained while following the advice in this book.

An Hachette UK Company
www.hachette.co.uk

First published in Great Britain in 2017 by Spruce,
a division of Octopus Publishing Group Ltd, Carmelite House,
50 Victoria Embankment, London, EC4Y 0DZ
www.octopusbooks.co.uk
www.octopusbooksusa.com

Copyright © Octopus Publishing Group Ltd 2017

Distributed in the US by Hachette Book Group,
1290 Avenue of the Americas, 4th and 5th Floors, New York, NY 10104

Distributed in Canada by Canadian Manda Group
664 Annette Street, Toronto, Ontario, Canada M6S 2C8

This material was previously published as *Miracle Juices: Immune Boosters*

ISBN 978-1-84601-543-4

A CIP catalogue record for this book is available
from the British Library

Printed and bound in China

10 9 8 7 6 5 4 3 2 1

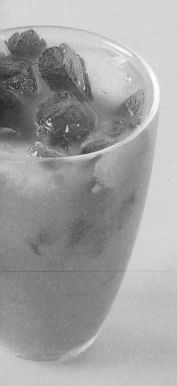

Contents

introduction

Is your immune system suffering?

Do you catch every bug that is being passed around the office or at home? Are you always sniffling and sneezing? If the answer is yes, your biggest ally in the fight against sickness is a strong immune system. Building up your immunity will not only help you resist disease now, but also lower your chances of suffering from chronic illnesses in later life.

We are surrounded by germs every day of our lives and the human body can be very resourceful in dealing with them. It has a whole host of tricks to fight off viruses, bacteria and other unwanted visitors. But if you aren't eating a balanced diet containing the correct proportions of certain vitamins and minerals, then the immune system will take a tumble, and all those germs will be able to get a hold on the body.

How the immune system works

- The skin, stomach acid, friendly bacteria in the gut, urine and tears act as a first line of defence against unwanted germs.
- White blood cells called lymphocytes travel around the body on the look out for any bacteria, viruses or other infecting agents. Once they have found a foreign body, they produce antibodies and toxins that will exterminate it.
- Monocytes and macrophages (other forms of white blood cells) encompass any germs that are found and digest them. You will know this is happening when inflammation occurs.

How to boost the immune system

There are ten key nutrients which really have an effect on boosting the immune system: vitamin A, beta-carotene, vitamin B complex, vitamin C, vitamin E, calcium, selenium, zinc, iron and magnesium. Collectively, they support the immune system by:

- Acting as powerful antioxidants, antiviral and antibacterial agents, and antihistamines. Antioxidants protect the body against damage by free radicals, which can cause degenerative disease.
- Maintaining the lymphatic system and helping in the production of white blood cells and antibodies.
- Helping convert essential fatty acids into anti-inflammatory prostaglandins. Without prostaglandins, the body couldn't regulate the activity of the white blood cells, which would lead to more colds, infections and allergies.
- Guarding against the damage caused by pollution.

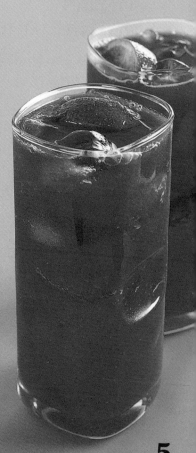

phytonutrients

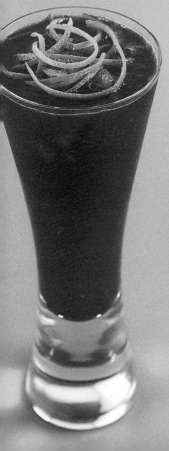

Recent research has unearthed a whole new set of compounds that, although not classed as essential to life, can have a very positive impact on our health. These are known as phytonutrients and there are well over a hundred different types.

They are powerful antioxidants that work hand in hand with vitamins and minerals to keep degenerative diseases at bay and maintain a healthy immune system.

The simplest way to ensure you are preparing food rich in these compounds is to include naturally colourful fruits, vegetables and even seaweed in your diet.

Where to find phytonutrients

- Lycopene is found in red food, primarily tomatoes.
- Curcumin is present in yellow food, such as corn and yellow peppers.
- Anthoxanthins are also found in yellow foods. Potatoes and yellow-skinned onions are good sources.
- Carotenoids are of particular benefit to the immune system. Any foods in the orange spectrum will provide them. Eat plenty of cantaloupe melon, papaya, mangoes, carrots, apricots and squash.

- Anthocyanidins and proanthocyanidins come cloaked in the colours purple or blue. Raise your intake of blueberries, blackberries, black cherries, black grapes, blackcurrants, beetroot and cranberries.

- Chlorophyll promotes quick healing and guards against diseases such as cancer. Wherever you see green, you'll find it. Include some of these every day: cabbage, broccoli, kale, salad leaves, seaweed, wheatgrass and algae such as spirulina.

top tips

- The B vitamins and vitamin C readily dissolve in water, so when cooking vegetables or brown rice, use the cooking water in the finished meal as it is a concentrated source of vitamins.
- Drink fresh juices soon after making them as many vitamins degrade quickly on contact with air.
- Vitamins A and C are easily perishable in the human body, so your intake should be spread throughout the day for maximum benefit.
- Key sources of antioxidants are all orange, red, purple, yellow and green fruits and vegetables, potatoes, nuts, seeds, wheatgerm, garlic and onions, shellfish, poultry, whole grains, liver, eggs, lean meat and full-fat dairy produce.
- Key sources of essential fatty acids include cold-pressed oils, nuts, seeds and oily fish.
- In a world where food processing is sapping the goodness out of wholesome natural foods and our eating habits leave a lot to be desired, vitamin and mineral supplements may be required. Always consult a qualified nutritionist to identify what you may be lacking before embarking on a supplement program.

top ten nutrients

Nutrient	Actions	Best Source	Recommended daily dosage
Vitamin A	Antioxidant; metabolizes fatty acids; fight colds and infections; maintains mucous membranes; maintains the thymus gland.	Liver, eggs, full-fat dairy produce, cod liver oil, oily fish.	4000–10,000 iu
Beta-carotene	Converted into vitamin A in the body.	Butternut squash, pumpkin, melon, sweet potatoes, carrots, apricots, mangoes, green leafy vegetables.	4000–10000 iu
Vitamin B complex	Vitamins B6 and B3 help convert essential fatty acids into anti-inflammatory prostaglandins. B5 is required for antibody production and maintains the white blood cells.	Whole grains, liver, poultry, game, wheatgerm, brewers yeast.	B1: 1.5 mg, B2: 1.7 mg, B3: 20 mg, B6: 2 mg, B12: 6 mcg
Vitamin C	Helps absorb calcium, iron and certain amino acids; enables the body to excrete poisonous substances; increases immune response; has antihistamine properties; helps prevent anaemia; speeds up the healing process of wounds; a powerful antioxidant.	Broccoli, parsley, kiwi fruit, citrus fruit, berries, peppers, blackcurrants, Brussels sprouts, papaya, mangoes.	100 mg minimum. Many nutritionists recommend 1500–4000 mg
Vitamin E	Powerful antioxidant; helps pituitary hormone production; assists cellular regeneration; guards against pollutants; accelerates healing; inhibits carcinogens; helps antibody response to infection.	Avocado, nuts, seeds, unrefined oils, wheatgerm, oatmeal.	12–15 iu minimum. 100–600 iu is recommended by nutritionists.

Nutrient	Actions	Best Source	Recommended daily dosage
Calcium	Vital for the bones and phagocytic cells; helps the metabolism of essential fatty acids.	Dairy products, fortified soya products, nuts, seeds, tinned fish with bones, dark green vegetables.	800–1200 mg
Magnesium	Activates metabolic enzymes; helps utilize vitamins C and E; helps convert glucose to energy; necessary for antibody production.	Nuts, seeds, green leafy vegetables, root vegetables, egg yolks, whole grains, dried fruit.	350–450 mg
Iron	Vital for formation of haemoglobin and white blood cells and antibodies; relieves fatigue; prevents anaemia; promotes immune system; and aids growth.	Liver, red meat, eggs, whole grains, green leafy vegetables, beans, lentils, nuts, seeds, blackstrap molasses.	10–18 mg
Zinc	Essential for the immune system; vital for the production of white blood cells, especially the lymphocytes; metabolizes essential fatty acids; lowers histamine production; accelerates healing; helps form insulin; increases overall natural immunity.	Shellfish, poultry, game, lean red meat, pulses, seeds, nuts, whole grains.	15–40 mg
Selenium	A powerful antioxidant; helps in the production of antibodies.	Nuts, seeds, whole grains, seafood.	50–200 mcg

why juice?

Vital vitamins and minerals such as antioxidants, vitamins A, B, C and E, folic acid, potassium, calcium, magnesium, zinc and amino acids are present in fresh fruits and vegetables, and are all necessary for optimum health. Because juicing removes the indigestible fibre in fruits and vegetables, the nutrients are available to the body in much larger quantities than if the piece of fruit or vegetable were eaten whole. For example, when you eat a raw carrot you are able to assimilate only about 1 per cent of the available beta-carotene, because many of the nutrients are trapped in the fibre. When a carrot is juiced, thereby removing the fibre, nearly 100 per cent of the beta-carotene can be assimilated. Juicing several types of fruits and vegetables on a daily basis is therefore an easy way to ensure that your body receives its full quota of vitamins and minerals.

In addition, fruits and vegetables provide another substance absolutely essential for good health — water.

Most people don't consume enough water. In fact, many of the fluids we drink — coffee, tea, soft drinks, alcoholic beverages and artificially flavoured drinks — contain substances that require extra water for the body to eliminate, and tend to be dehydrating. Fruit and vegetable juices are free of these unnecessary substances.

Your health
A diet high in fruits and vegetables can prevent and help to cure a wide range of ailments. At the cutting edge of nutritional research are the plant chemicals known as phytochemicals, which hold the key to preventing deadly diseases such as cancer and heart disease, and others such as asthma, arthritis and allergies.

Although juicing benefits your overall health, it should be used only to complement your daily eating plan. You must still eat enough from the other food groups (such as grains, dairy food and pulses) to ensure your body maintains strong bones and healthy cells. If you are following a specially prescribed diet, or are under medical supervision, do discuss any drastic changes with your health practitioner before beginning any type of new health regime.

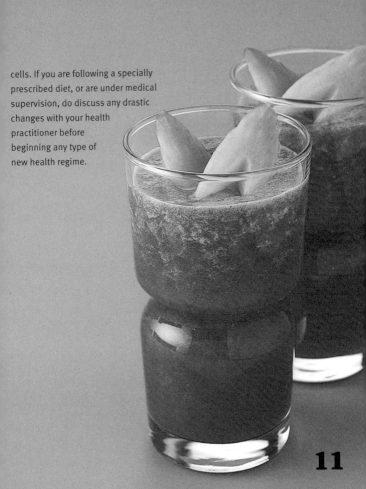

how to juice

Available in a variety of models, juicers work by separating the fruit and vegetable juice from the pulp. Choose a juicer with a reputable brand name, that has an opening big enough for larger fruits and vegetables, and make sure it is easy to take apart and clean, otherwise you may become discouraged from using it.

Types of juicer

A citrus juicer, or lemon squeezer is ideal for extracting the juice from oranges, lemons, limes and grapefruit, especially if you want to add just a small amount of citrus juice to another liquid. Pure citrus juice has a high acid content, which may upset or irritate your stomach, so is best diluted with water.

Centrifugal juicers are the most widely used and affordable juicers on the market. Fresh fruits and vegetables are fed into a rapidly spinning grater, and the pulp separated from the juice by centrifugal force. The pulp is retained in the machine while the juice runs into a separate jug. A centrifugal juicer produces less juice than the more expensive masticating juicer, which works by pulverizing fruits and vegetables and pushing them through a wire mesh with immense force.

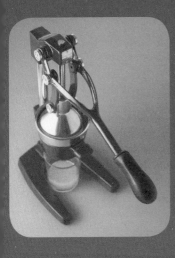

Preparing produce for juicing

Prepare ingredients just before juicing so that fewer nutrients are lost through oxidization. Cut or tear foods into manageable pieces for juicing. If the ingredients are not organic, do not include stems, skins or roots, but if the produce is organic, you can put everything in the juicer. However, don't include the skins from pineapple, mango, papaya, citrus fruit and banana, and remove the stones from avocados, apricots, peaches, mangoes and plums. You can include melon seeds, particularly watermelon, as these are full of juice. For grape juice, choose green grapes with an amber tinge or black grapes with a darkish bloom. Leave the pith on lemons for the pectin content.

Cleaning the juicer

Clean your juicing machine thoroughly – a toothbrush or nailbrush works well for removing stubborn residual pulp. Soaking the equipment in warm soapy water will loosen the residue from those hard-to-reach places. A solution of one part white vinegar to two parts water will lessen any staining from the fruits and vegetables.

13

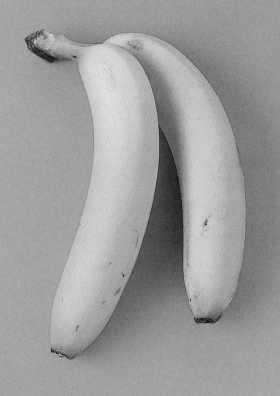

heal

This drink is bursting with beta-carotene, which is converted into vitamin A in the body.

lift-off

100 g (3½ oz) red pepper
125 g (4 oz) strawberries
50 g (2 oz) tomato
125 g (4 oz) mango
125 g (4 oz) watermelon
3 ice cubes
mango slices, to decorate
  (optional)

Juice all the ingredients, whizz in a blender or food processor with the ice cubes and serve in a tall glass. Decorate with mango slices, if liked.
Makes 200 ml (7 fl oz)

Nutritional Values

- Kcals: 200
- vitamin A: 9630 iu
- vitamin C: 231 mg
- selenium: 2.66 mcg
- zinc: 0.58 mg

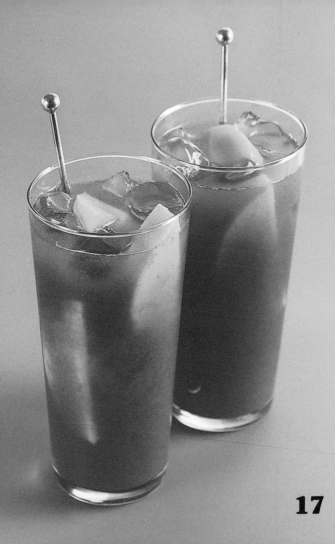

17

Spinach is a useful source of iron. It also contains good amounts of vitamins C, E, B1 and B6, and folic acid.

get up and go

large handful of baby spinach
200 g (7 oz) carrot
4 tomatoes
½ red pepper
ice cubes

Juice the vegetables in alternating batches to ensure the spinach leaves do not clog the juicer. Pour the juice into a glass and add a couple of ice cubes.
Makes 300 ml (½ pint)

Nutritional Values

- Kcals: 175
- vitamin A: 71065 iu
- vitamin C: 208 mg
- vitamin E: 3.33 mg
- iron: 3.8 mg
- calcium: 169 mg

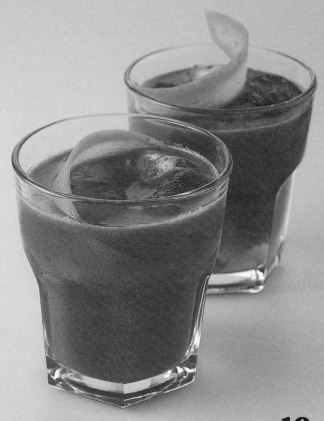

19

This juice is packed with vitamin B3, niacin and folic acid.

green dream

250 g (8 oz) apple
50 g (2 oz) celery
50 g (2 oz) kiwi fruit
½ lemon
100 g (3 ½ oz) avocado

Juice the apple, celery, kiwi fruit and lemon. Transfer to a blender with the avocado and whizz for 20 seconds. Decorate with kiwi slices if liked.
Makes 200 ml (7 fl oz)

Nutritional Values

- Kcals: 347
- vitamin C 161 mg
- vitamin E 2.89 mg
- niacin 2.42 mg
- folic acid 72 mg

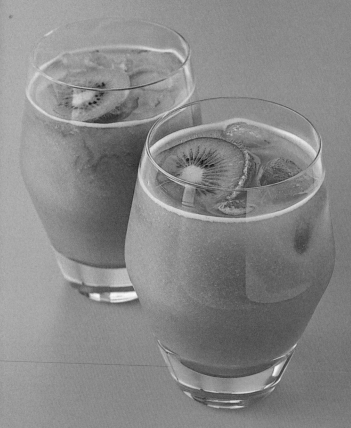

A juice rich in antioxidants. The lime encourages the elimination of toxins.

ginger zinger

125 g (4 oz) carrot
250 g (8 oz) cantaloupe
melon
1 lime
2.5 cm (1 inch) cube
fresh root ginger,
roughly chopped
ice cubes

To decorate:
lime wedges
cardamom seeds

Juice the carrot, melon, lime and ginger.
Serve in a glass over ice. Decorate
with lime wedges and seeds from a
cardamom pod.
Makes 200 ml (7 fl oz)

Nutritional Values

- Kcals: 166
- vitamin A: 4262 iu
- vitamin C: 137 mg
- selenium: 2.7 mcg
- zinc: 0.84 mg

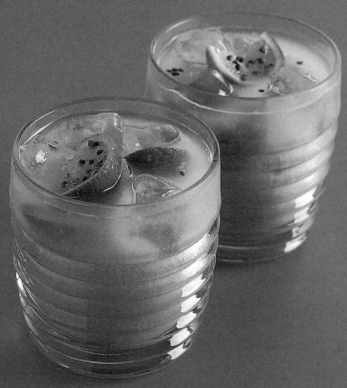

23

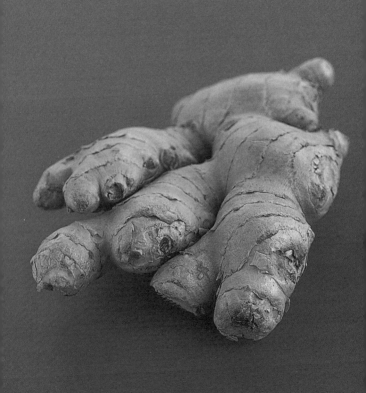

fortify

Papaya helps to calm the digestive system; cucumber flushes out toxins and orange gives a great boost of vitamin C. The overall effect is calming and rehydrating.

morning after

125 g (4 oz) papaya
2 oranges
125 g (4 oz) cucumber
ice cubes

To decorate:
cucumber slices
papaya slices

Peel the papaya and the oranges, leaving on as much pith as possible. Juice them together with the cucumber and serve in a tall glass over ice. Decorate with slices of cucumber and papaya.
Makes 200 ml (7 fl oz)

Nutritional Values

- Kcals: 184
- vitamin A: 1123 iu
- vitamin C: 218 mg
- magnesium: 51 mg
- potassium: 1004 mg
- selenium: 2 mcg

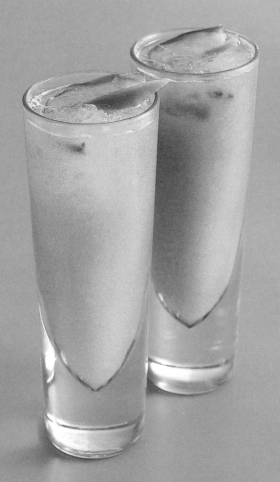

27

The magnesium in the parsley has a calming effect; it is also present in celery.
Garlic is renowned for its antibacterial, antibiotic, antiseptic and antiviral properties.

root 66

175 g (6 oz) carrot
175 g (6 oz) parsnip
175 g (6 oz) celery sticks
175 g (6 oz) sweet potato
a handful of parsley
1 garlic clove

Juice all the ingredients together and whizz in a blender with 2 ice cubes. Serve in a wide glass decorated with a wedge of lemon and a parsley sprig, if liked.
Makes 200 ml (7 fl oz)

Nutritional Values

- Kcals: 386
- vitamin A 51,192 iu
- vitamin C 136.35 mg
- potassium 2,882.5 mg
- magnesium 150.5 mg

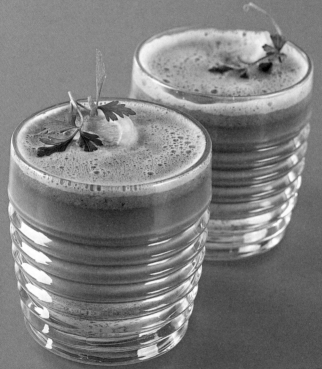

29

This juice is another good choice if you're run down and fighting the winter round of colds and flu. Peppers are a favourite for warding off infection, and are also natural painkillers.

sergeant pep-up

1 orange
100 g (3½ oz) red pepper
100 g (3½ oz) yellow
   pepper
100 g (3½ oz) orange
   pepper
ice cubes
1 tablespoon mint leaves,
   plus extra to decorate

Peel the orange, leaving on as much pith as possible. Juice the peppers and orange and serve in a tumbler with ice cubes. Stir in the mint and decorate with mint leaves, if liked.

Makes 200 ml (7 fl oz)

Nutritional Values

- Kcals: 141
- vitamin A: 2146 iu
- vitamin C: 333 mg
- selenium: 1.52 mcg
- zinc: 0.44 mg

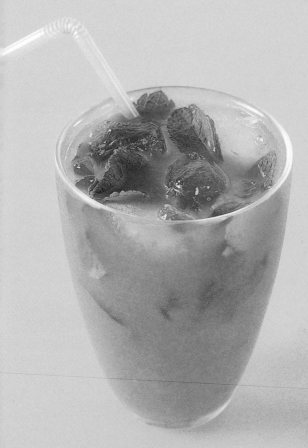

A sweet dairy-free milk shake that aids digestion and is full of protein, calcium and vitamin C.

super
shakey

250 g (8 oz) pineapple
100 g (3 ½ oz) parsnip
100 g (3 ½ oz) carrot
5 tablespoons soy milk

Juice the pineapple, parsnip and carrot. Whizz in a blender with the soy milk and a couple of ice cubes. Decorate with pineapple wedges if liked.
Makes 200 ml (7 fl oz)

Nutritional Values

- Kcals: 266
- vitamin C 65 mg
- calcium 80 mg
- protein 6 g

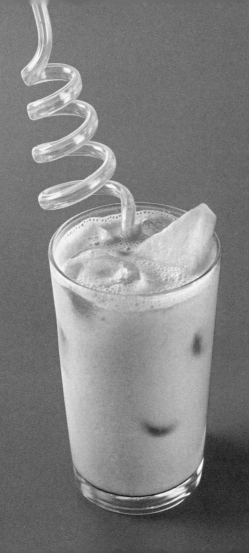

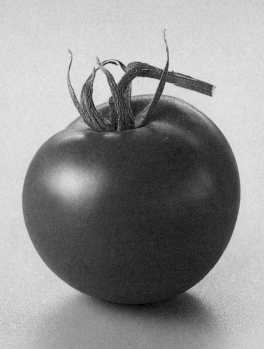

protect

This juice is rich in vitamin C, which is great for fighting off bronchial illness. Enzymes in the pineapple dissolve mucus, and the chilli is a great expectorant. Chillies are rich in carotenoids and vitamin C, and are thought to help increase blood flow. They also have antibacterial properties, which make them a favourite for beating colds and flu.

chill buster

250 g (8 oz) carrot
½ small deseeded chilli
    or a sprinkling of chilli
    powder
250 g (8 oz) pineapple
ice cubes
½ lime
1 tablespoon chopped
    coriander leaves

Juice the carrot, chilli and pineapple. Serve in a tall glass over ice cubes. Squeeze in the lime juice and stir in the chopped coriander leaves to serve.
Makes 200 ml (7 fl oz)

Nutritional Values

- Kcals: 240
- vitamin A: 70382 iu
- vitamin C: 72 mg
- selenium: 3.95 mcg
- zinc: 0.73 mg

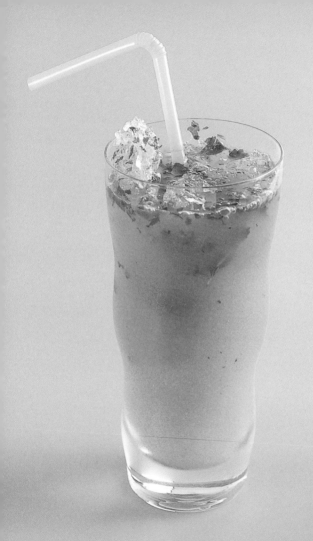

37

If you're run down and haven't been eating a balanced diet, your immune system becomes more susceptible to colds and flu. At the first sign of symptoms, drinking juices with papaya, lemon, lime, garlic or ginger may help.

frisky sour

150 g (5 oz) papaya
150 g (5 oz) grapefruit
150 g (5 oz) raspberries
½ lime
ice cubes
lime slices, to decorate

Scoop out the flesh of the papaya, and juice it with the grapefruit (with the pith left on), and the raspberries. Squeeze in the lime juice and mix. Serve with a few ice cubes and decorate with lime slices.
Makes 200 ml (7 fl oz)

Nutritional Values

- Kcals: 193
- vitamin A: 810 iu
- vitamin C: 188 mg
- selenium: 4.05 mcg
- zinc: 1.09 mg

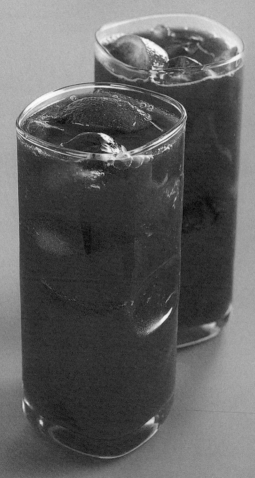

Tomatoes and carrots provide large amounts of vitamin C, ideal for maintaining a healthy body. Garlic, ginger and horseradish are all powerful antioxidants – imperative for fighting off infections. Combined, they also deal a mighty anti-mucus punch.

hot stuff

300 g (10 oz) tomato
100 g (3½ oz) celery
2.5 cm (1 inch) cube
  fresh root ginger,
  roughly chopped
1 garlic clove
2.5 cm (1 inch) cube
  fresh horseradish
175 g (6 oz) carrot
2 ice cubes
celery slivers, to decorate
  (optional)

Juice all the ingredients, whizz the juice in a blender or food processor with the ice cubes and serve in a tumbler. Decorate with celery slivers, if liked.
Makes 150 ml (¼ pint)

Nutritional Values

- Kcals: 189
- vitamin A: 51253 iu
- vitamin C: 87 mg
- selenium: 4.47 mcg
- zinc: 5.52 mg

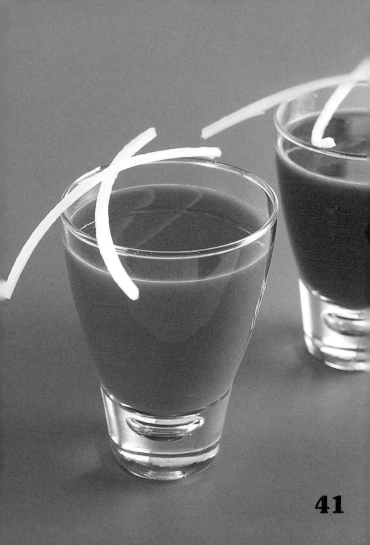

This simple and quenching juice is bursting with vitamin C and betacarotene, making it an invaluable immune booster.

red-hot remedy

4 large tomatoes
1 apple
1 celery stick
ice cubes
4 basil leaves, finely
   chopped
1½ tablespoons lime juice

Juice the tomatoes, apple and celery. Pour into a glass over ice, and stir in the basil and lime juice.
Makes 200 ml (7 fl oz)

Nutritional Values

- Kcals: 203
- vitamin A: 5718 iu
- magnesium: 63 mg
- zinc: 0.6 mg

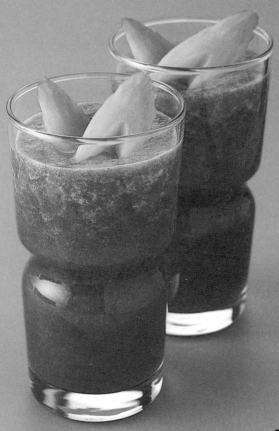

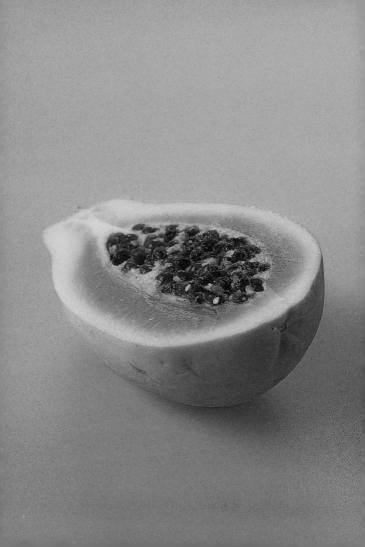

defend

This juice is full of vitamin C and phytonutrients, such as anthocyanidins, to help resist disease.

tummy tickler

300 g (10 oz) apple
200 g (7 oz)
   blackcurrants
ice cubes

Juice the fruit and serve over ice for a great blackcurrant cordial substitute. Decorate with extra blackcurrants, if liked.
Makes 200 ml (7 fl oz)

Nutritional Values

- Kcals: 300
- vitamin C: 415 mg
- calcium: 30 mg

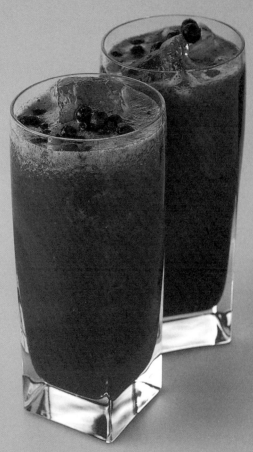

47

Peach has an alkalizing effect on the digestive system, and ginger works wonders for nausea.

peach fizz

250 g (8 oz) peach
2.5 cm (1 inch) cube
   fresh root ginger,
   roughly chopped
sparkling mineral water
mint leaves

Juice the peach and ginger and serve in a tall glass over ice, with a splash of sparkling water and a couple of mint leaves. Sip slowly to calm your stomach.
Makes 200 ml (7 fl oz)

Nutritional Values

- Kcals: 127
- vitamin C 10 mg
- potassium 390 mg

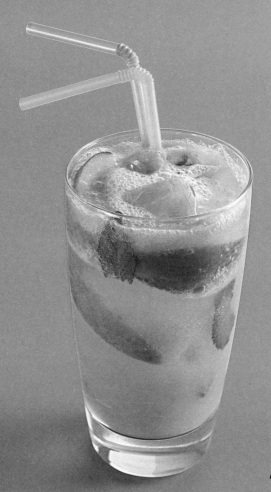

49

This juice packs a mighty antiviral punch, as it is bursting with vitamin C.

calm seas

2 oranges
1 kiwi fruit
200 g (7 oz) strawberries

Peel the oranges, leaving on as much pith as possible. Juice the oranges, kiwi fruit and strawberries, reserving some strawberries for decoration. Serve immediately.
Makes 200 ml (7 fl oz)

Nutritional Values

- Kcals: 201
- vitamin A: 726 iu
- vitamin C: 403 mg
- magnesium: 70 mg
- zinc: 0.8 mg

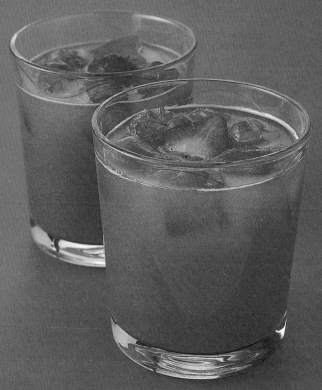

Full of iron, calcium and potassium, this is an all-round booster that is great for bones and teeth and keeping colds at bay.

top
banana

100 g (3½ oz) orange
150 g (5 oz) carrot
100 g (3½ oz) banana
1 dried apricot
ice cubes
banana chunks, to
**   decorate (optional)**

Peel the orange, leaving on as much pith as possible. Juice the carrot and orange. Whizz in a blender or food processor with the banana, apricot and some ice cubes. Decorate with chunks of banana, if liked.

Makes 200 ml (7 fl oz)

Nutritional Values

- Kcals: 204
- vitamin A: 44570 iu
- vitamin C: 88 mg
- calcium: 101 mg
- potassium: 1475 mg
- iron: 2.5 mg

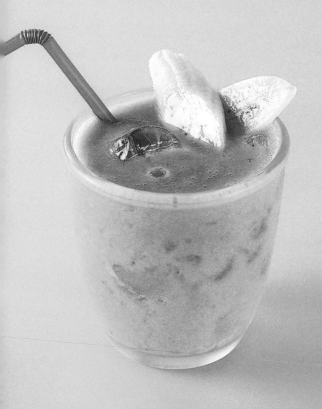

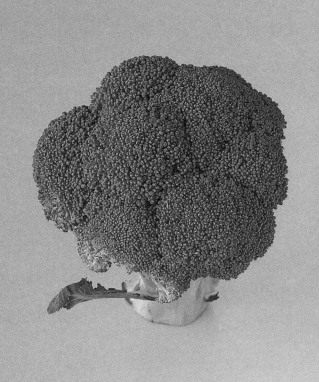

strengthen

This juice is an excellent source of vitamins A, C, B1, B6 and potassium. In addition to being a natural remedy for travel sickness and morning sickness, ginger is also believed to aid digestion and help the body fight off colds.

pick-me-up

200 g (7 oz) carrot
1 tart-flavoured apple,
such as Granny Smith
1 cm (½ inch) cube fresh
root ginger
ice cubes

Juice the carrots with the apple and ginger. Pour into a glass and add a couple of ice cubes.
Makes 250 ml (8 fl oz)

Nutritional Values

- Kcals: 127
- vitamin A: 60833 iu
- vitamin C: 30 mg
- iron: 0.9 mg
- calcium: 59 mg

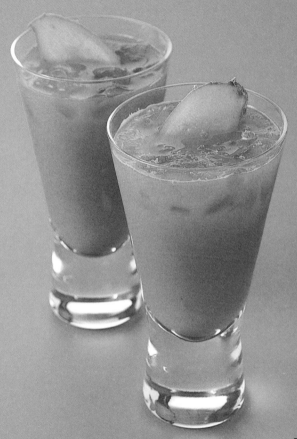

High in selenium, this is an ideal juice for smokers as it helps guard against lung cancer.

what's up broc?

**250 g (8 oz) broccoli
175 g (6 oz) carrot
50 g (2 oz) beetroot
coriander sprig, to
    decorate (optional)**

Juice all the ingredients and serve in a tall glass. Decorate with a coriander sprig, if liked.
Makes 200 ml (7 fl oz)

Nutritional Values

- Kcals: 172
- vitamin A: 52304 iu
- vitamin C: 43 mg
- selenium: 9.86 mcg
- zinc: 1.6 mg

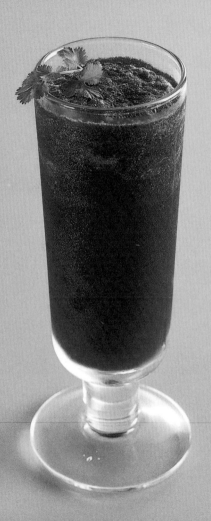

59

This juice is full of vitamins A and C, which should help keep colds at bay. Citrus fruits are also great mucus reducers.

vitamin vitality

2 oranges
125 g (4 oz) carrot

Peel the oranges, leaving on as much pith as possible. Juice the carrots with the oranges. Serve immediately.
Makes 200 ml (7 fl oz)

Nutritional Values

- Kcals: 188
- vitamin A: 34293 iu
- vitamin C: 151 mg
- magnesium: 44 mg
- zinc: 0.4 mg

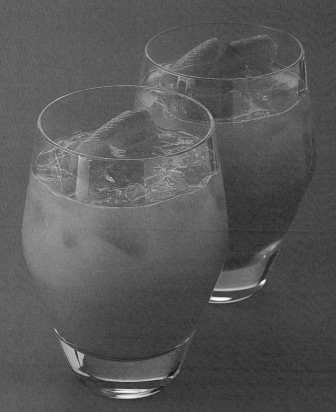

This juice has a high vitamin C content to ward off colds.
Strawberries are natural painkillers.

strawberry soother

200 g (7 oz) orange
200 g (7 oz) strawberries
ice cubes

Peel the orange, leaving on as much pith as possible. Juice the strawberries and orange, reserving some strawberries for decoration. Serve straight over ice, or whizz in a blender or food processor with a couple of ice cubes for a thicker drink.
Makes 200 ml (7 fl oz)

Nutritional Values

- Kcals: 154
- vitamin C: 219 mg
- potassium: 694 mg
- calcium: 108 mg

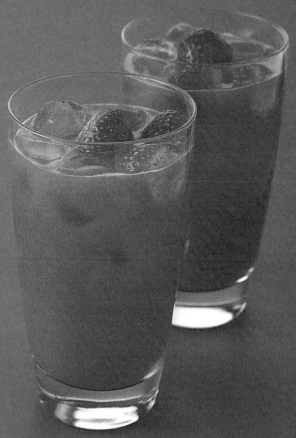

index

acknowledgements

The publisher would like to thank The Juicer Company
for the loan of the Champion juicer and the Orange X
citrus juicer (featured on pages 12 and 13).

Executive Editor Nicola Hill
Editor Camilla James
Executive Art Editor Geoff Fennell
Designer Sue Michniewicz
Senior Production Controller Jo Sim
Photographer Stephen Conroy
Home Economist David Morgan
Stylist Angela Swaffield
All photographs © Octopus
Publishing Group Ltd

DETOX

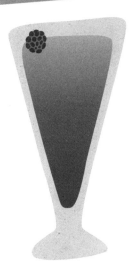

spruce

An Hachette UK Company
www.hachette.co.uk

First published in Great Britain in 2017 by Spruce,
a division of Octopus Publishing Group Ltd, Carmelite House,
50 Victoria Embankment, London, EC4Y 0DZ
www.octopusbooks.co.uk
www.octopusbooksusa.com

Copyright © Octopus Publishing Group Ltd 2017

Distributed in the US by Hachette Book Group,
1290 Avenue of the Americas, 4th and 5th Floors, New York, NY 10104

Distributed in Canada by Canadian Manda Group
664 Annette Street, Toronto, Ontario, Canada M6S 2C8

This material was previously published as *Miracle Juices: Detox*

ISBN 978-1-84601-543-4

A CIP catalogue record for this book is available
from the British Library

Printed and bound in China

10 9 8 7 6 5 4 3 2 1

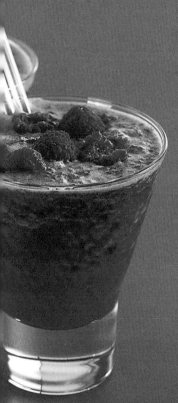

Contents

introduction

The case for detox

Modern life is necessarily toxic to some extent. Every day we face a multitude of pollutants and chemicals in the air that we breathe and in the food and water we consume. In addition, we tend to run our lives at an incredible pace — we have demanding, stressful jobs that may involve long hours of travelling, we run homes, bring up children and usually try to fit in hectic social lives, too. Because time is short, we invariably cut corners. We eat convenience or junk food, we don't get enough sleep or exercise and we often smoke or drink too much alcohol as a quick-fix way to relax.

The body treats all the toxins it encounters as a matter of urgency and works on processing them to render them harmless, or 'detoxed'.

This leaves less energy for the everyday processes of cleansing, healing and renewal. Over time, the body can't keep up the pace, the strain shows on the overworked liver and kidneys and the body's performance slows down. The effects of this slow-down and the build-up of toxins emerge in many different forms — everything from continual fatigue, passing infections, skin eruptions, headaches and digestive problems to serious conditions, such as ulcers, cancer and heart disease.

How detox works

A detoxification diet allows two things to happen. First, by abstaining from certain foods we stop overloading the body with harmful substances and, secondly, we give it plenty of the right nutrients to actually speed up the elimination of old toxins and unwanted waste and promote cell renewal. As the cells are rejuvenated, your body becomes healthier and you look and feel younger! As well as losing any excess weight, you can expect to have clear skin, healthy-looking hair, strong nails and lots more energy. Detoxing also has a very calming effect on the mind, particularly if you combine it with a relaxation technique, such as yoga or meditation.

Detoxification need not involve only diet. There are various external treatments that can work alongside a detox diet to help the general detox process. These include facial exfoliation, hydrotherapy, skin brushing and manual lymphatic drainage massage.

detox guidelines

A detoxification programme is ideal if you have been over-indulging and feel lethargic, listless and bloated. Don't attempt a lengthy detox programme, which you may break early out of sheer hunger. Instead, try a weekend-long detox plan, or even a one-day juice plan (see pages 8–9), and concentrate on drinking juices that speed up the detox process and aid digestion and the immune system. A one-day detox can be repeated every week if you wish.

Since much of the nutritional value of food is lost in its cooking and processing, uncooked fresh produce with its high vitamin and mineral content is at the core of any detox plan. A one-day detox plan consists entirely of freshly made fruit and vegetable juices, which help cleanse the blood and tissues of toxins and regenerate the entire system. Organic fresh produce is preferable so that you don't replace some of the toxins you are eliminating with pesticide residues.

A longer detox programme involves several stages, starting with liquids only, then gradually adding raw fruits and vegetables, cooked vegetables and brown rice, grains and live yogurts, and finally fish. After any period of consuming liquids only you must return to food slowly or you will overload the digestive system, undo all you have achieved and even feel unwell.

During detoxification, side effects such as tiredness, muscle pains, mood swings, headaches and skin problems are inevitable as the toxins make their way out. However, do persevere — within a relatively short time you will feel re-energized and rejuvenated, and have better-looking skin, hair and nails.

Do not detox if you:
- are underweight
- are pregnant or breast-feeding
- have anaemia
- have Type 1 diabetes
- are following a course of prescription medication
- have kidney failure
- have severe liver disease

After detox

By eliminating the substances that are harmful to your body — in particular caffeine, nicotine, alcohol, over-the-counter drugs (but check with your doctor about prescribed drugs) and processed carbohydrates and sugars — your body will feel lighter and less bloated. Continue the good work after detoxing by keeping your intake of these substances moderate or banishing them from your diet altogether and replacing them with healthy alternatives.

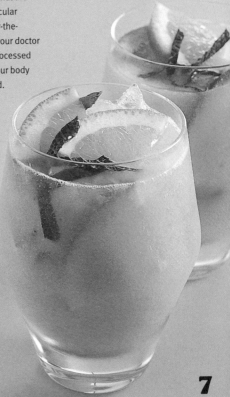

one-day detox plan

A one-day juice detox is beneficial for two reasons. You'll be clearing your body of a build-up of toxins, which could be contributing to certain ailments. Also, although you may feel slightly tired or headachy as your body goes without sugars or caffeine, it should be a day dedicated solely to you,

8.00 am	Drink a glass of warm water with a little lemon juice to help flush out the kidneys.
8.30 am	Make a juice with a little citrus fruit in it, or apple, pineapple or melon (*see* Ultimate Detox, page 18, 'C' Red, page 36, or Pure Cure, page 52) to wake you up and begin the cleansing process.
9.00 am	Get your circulation moving with dry skin brushing to stimulate the circulatory and lymphatic systems. Using a natural bristle brush, begin at your feet, and with long, smooth movements gently move upwards. Finish with a warm shower then a blast of cold water if you're feeling brave! Dry yourself and moisturize your skin.
9.30 am	Have a glass of water or a herbal tea which will aid the detox process.
10.00 am	Take a gentle walk or swim or try a yoga class. By moving your body, you're less likely to feel the side effects of a detox, such as tiredness or headaches, and you'll also be helping your body rid itself of toxins.
11.30 am	After exercising, have another glass of water or a herbal tea.
12.30 pm	At lunchtime, choose a filling juice to alleviate hunger pains. Try a combination of root vegetables and leafy greens (*see* Green Peace, page 16, or Squeaky Green, page 56).
1.00pm	Have another glass of water or a herbal tea — ginger is good for the stomach, while lemon is a good tea for detoxification.

to relax and rejuvenate. Try not to arrange any appointments and, if you want to exercise, don't do anything too strenuous. Do something you enjoy, whether it's reading, relaxing or having a lie-in. There are no hard and fast rules for a one-day detox, just spend the day looking after yourself.

1.30pm	A detox programme can be quite tiring, as your body is ridding itself of a build-up of toxins. Have a nap or lie down and read or listen to some relaxing music.
2.30pm	Have another glass of water or a herbal tea.
3.30pm	Your blood sugar levels may be feeling a little low by now, so you can pack this juice full of fruits such as blueberries, strawberries, cranberries, oranges and mangoes. It may taste slightly tart after a relatively food-free day, but you'll feel energized afterwards.
5.00pm	It's important to drink at least eight glasses of water every day, so have another glass now.
7.30pm	You'll probably have no problems going to sleep tonight, but make a juice that contains ingredients such as bananas, lettuce or apples to aid relaxation and beat insomnia (*see* Fig Feast, page 28, or Sleep Tight, page 46).
9.30pm	Have another glass of water and then your last herbal tea, a calming one before bedtime, such as chamomile tea. Have a relaxing bath, adding aromatherapy oils such as lavender, ylang ylang, rose or sandalwood.
10.00pm	Bedtime. Your stomach will be relatively empty by tomorrow morning, so start the day gradually with some fresh fruit and yogurt or wholemeal toast and honey. Opt for a light salad lunch, and possibly some steamed vegetables and rice for dinner, supplemented of course by a couple of fresh nutritious juices.

9

why juice?

Vital vitamins and minerals such as antioxidants, vitamins A, B, C and E, folic acid, potassium, calcium, magnesium, zinc and amino acids are present in fresh fruits and vegetables, and are all necessary for optimum health. Because juicing removes the indigestible fibre in fruits and vegetables, the nutrients are available to the body in much larger quantities than if the piece of fruit or vegetable were eaten whole. For example, when you eat a raw carrot you are able to assimilate only about 1 per cent of the available beta-carotene, because many of the nutrients are trapped in the fibre. When a carrot is juiced, thereby removing the fibre, nearly 100 per cent of the beta-carotene can be assimilated. Juicing several types of fruits and vegetables on a daily basis is therefore an easy way to ensure that your body receives its full quota of vitamins and minerals.

In addition, fruits and vegetables provide another substance absolutely essential for good health — water. Most people don't consume enough water. In fact, many of the fluids we drink — coffee, tea, soft drinks, alcoholic beverages and artificially flavoured drinks — contain substances that require extra water for the body to eliminate, and tend to be dehydrating. Fruit and vegetable juices are free of these unnecessary substances.

Your health

A diet high in fruits and vegetables can prevent and help to cure a wide range of ailments. At the cutting edge of nutritional research are the plant chemicals known as phytochemicals, which hold the key to preventing deadly diseases such as cancer and heart disease, and others such as asthma, arthritis and allergies.

Although juicing benefits your overall health, it should be used only to complement your daily eating plan. You must still eat enough from the other food groups (such as grains, dairy food and pulses) to ensure your body maintains strong bones and healthy cells. If you are following a specially prescribed diet,

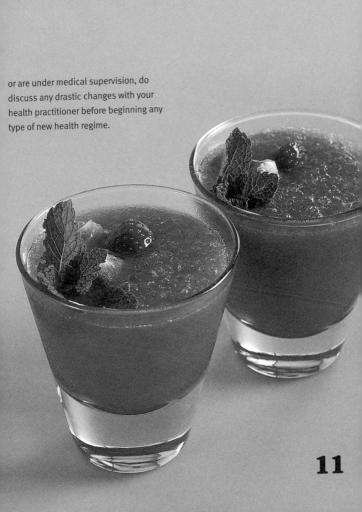

or are under medical supervision, do discuss any drastic changes with your health practitioner before beginning any type of new health regime.

11

how to juice

Available in a variety of models, juicers work by separating the fruit and vegetable juice from the pulp. Choose a juicer with a reputable brand name, that has an opening big enough for larger fruits and vegetables, and make sure it is easy to take apart and clean, otherwise you may become discouraged from using it.

Types of juicer

A citrus juicer or lemon squeezer is ideal for extracting the juice from oranges, lemons, limes and grapefruit, especially if you want to add just a small amount of citrus juice to another liquid. Pure citrus juice has a high acid content, which may upset your stomach, so it is best diluted.

Centrifugal juicers are the most widely used and affordable juicers available. Fresh fruits and vegetables are fed into a rapidly spinning grater, and the pulp separated from the juice by centrifugal force. The pulp is retained in the machine while the juice runs into a separate jug. A centrifugal juicer produces less juice than the more expensive masticating juicer, which works by pulverizing fruits and vegetables, and pushing them through a wire mesh with immense force.

Cleaning the juicer

Clean your juicing machine thoroughly, as any residue left may

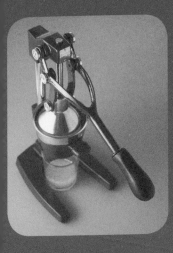

are lost through oxidization. Cut or tear foods into manageable pieces for juicing. If the ingredients are not organic, do not include stems, skins or roots, but if the produce is organic, you can put everything in the juicer. However, don't include the skins from pineapple, mango, papaya, citrus fruit and banana, and remove the stones from avocados, apricots, peaches, mangoes and plums. You can include melon seeds, particularly watermelon, as these are full of juice. For grape juice, choose green grapes with an amber tinge or black grapes with a darkish bloom. Leave the pith on lemons for the pectin content.

harbour bacterial growth -- a toothbrush or nailbrush works well for removing stubborn residual pulp. Leaving the equipment to soak in warm soapy water will loosen the residue from those hard-to-reach places. A solution made up of one part white vinegar to two parts water will lessen any staining produced by the fruits and vegetables.

Preparing produce for juicing
It is best to prepare ingredients just before juicing so that fewer nutrients

13

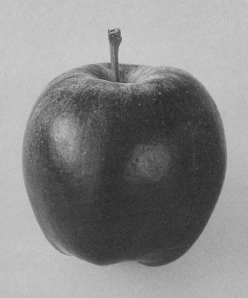

eliminate

A good detox juice, this ultra green juice helps to maintain energy levels. Leafy green vegetables are particularly good for an overtaxed liver. Parsley is a mild diuretic and contains zinc and trace minerals that aid liver function, while celery helps cleanse the liver and lymph system and aids digestion.

green peace

100 g (3½ oz) broccoli
100 g (3½ oz) kale
25 g (1 oz) parsley
200 g (7 oz) apple
50 g (2 oz) celery

Juice all the ingredients and serve in a glass over ice. Decorate with kale, if liked.
Makes 200 ml (7 fl oz)

Nutritional Values

- Kcals 228
- Vitamin A 10574 iu
- Vitamin C 365 mg
- Selenium 5.14 mcg
- Zinc 1 mg

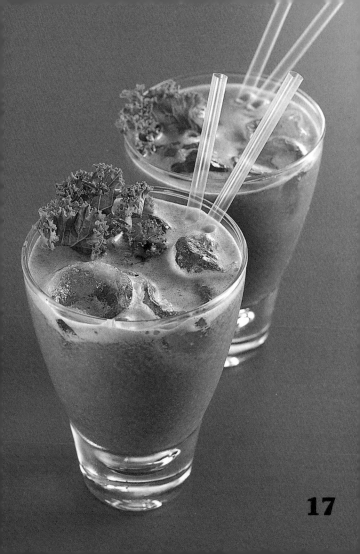

Simply delicious, this juice is the best general tonic for internal cleansing and for boosting the immune system. Both apples and carrots are exceptionally high in minerals and vitamins and are great cleansers.

ultimate detox

4 carrots
2 green apples

Juice both the ingredients and serve in a tall glass over ice. Decorate with slices of apple, if liked.
Makes 300 ml (½ pint)

Nutritional Values

- Kcals 280
- Vitamin A 80356 iu
- Vitamin C 44 mg
- Potassium 1280 mg

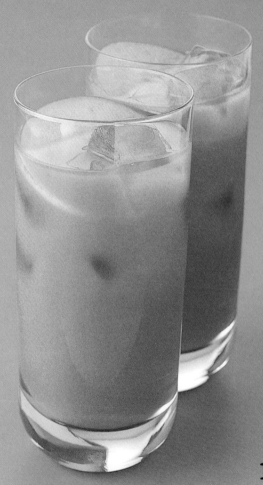

19

Watercress is a powerful cleansing detox ingredient, and pear can help to regulate bowel movement.

easy
does it

250 g (8 oz) pear
125 g (4 oz) watercress
½ lemon

Juice the ingredients and serve over ice. Add a twist of lemon, if liked.
Makes 50 ml (2 fl oz)

Nutritional Values

- Kcals 172
- vitamin A 5,935 iu
- vitamin C 85 mg
- calcium 185 mg
- vitamin B6 0.2 mg

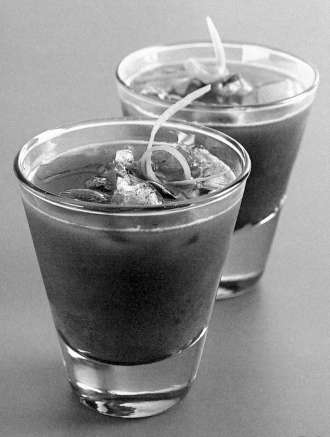

21

A diuretic, watermelon speeds the passage of fluids carrying toxins through the system. The seeds are full of juice and can be juiced too, if liked.

water baby

¼ watermelon, about 300 g (10 oz) flesh
125 g (4 oz) raspberries

Remove the skin from the watermelon and chop the flesh into even-sized pieces. Juice the watermelon and raspberries, pour into a large glass and add a couple of ice cubes. Decorate with raspberries, if liked.
Makes 350 ml (12 fl oz)

Nutritional Values

- Kcals 125
- Vitamin A 1330 iu
- Vitamin C 60 mg
- Potassium 559 mg
- Iron 1.8 mg
- Calcium 52 mg

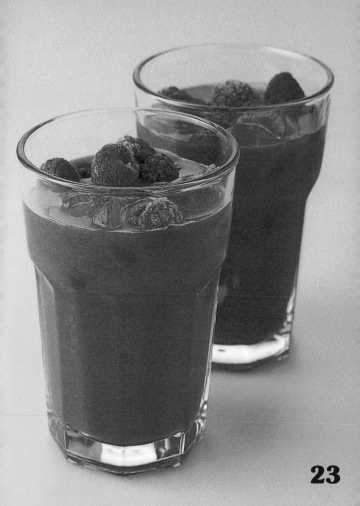

23

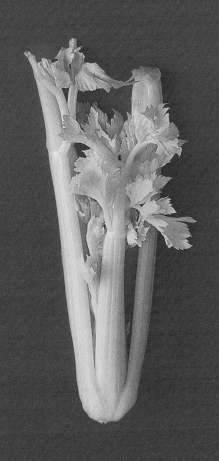

repair

The cucumber in this juice provides protective antioxidants for the digestive tract and, together with the melon and cranberries, acts as a diuretic to cleanse the intestinal system.

flush-a-bye-baby

250 g (8 oz) cranberries
250 g (8 oz) watermelon
   or galia melon, peeled
250 g (8 oz) cucumber

Juice all the ingredients, including the pips of the melon and the skin of the cucumber. Serve in a tumbler and decorate with melon sticks, if liked.
Makes 200 ml (7 fl oz)

Nutritional Values

- Kcals 232
- Vitamin A 8475 iu
- Vitamin C 120 mg
- Potassium 880 mg
- Iron 4.7 mg
- Calcium 92.5 mg

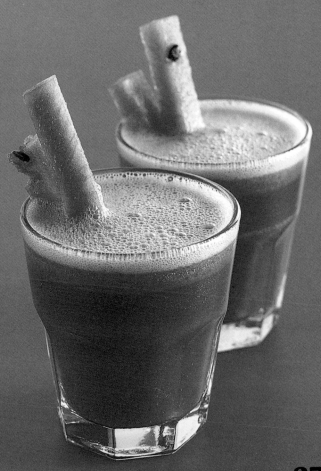

27

Bananas and figs are rich in tryptophan. This is converted in the body into the brain chemical serotonin, which can induce a feeling of wellbeing. Because these fruits are high in natural sugars they produce a feeling of fullness, which can help stave off hunger if you are on a juice-only detox plan.

fig feast

250 g (8 oz) carrot
100 g (3½ oz) figs
1 orange, peeled
2.5 cm (1 inch) cube
   of fresh root ginger,
   roughly chopped
100 g (3½ oz) peeled
   banana

Juice the carrot, figs, orange and ginger. Put the juice into a blender with the banana and a couple of ice cubes and whizz for 20 seconds for a delicious smoothie. Add more ice cubes and decorate with sliced figs, if liked.
Makes 200 ml (7 fl oz)

Nutritional Values

- Kcals 460
- Vitamin A 14117 iu
- Vitamin B6 0.23 mg
- Vitamin C 192 mg
- Magnesium 118 mg
- Tryptophan 89 mg

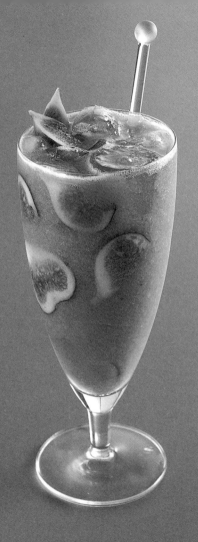

29

Cabbage is a great detoxifier. It aids digestion and prevents fluid retention and constipation. Cabbage is perfect for juicing as its nutrients are most abundant when it is eaten raw. Celery, watercress and pears are the ideal accompaniments as they also contribute to the detoxification process. Watercress is a powerful intestinal cleanser, the cabbage and the pear rid the colon of waste matter and the celery purifies the lymph.

spring clean

250 g (8 oz) pear
125 g (4 oz) cabbage
50 g (2 oz) celery
25 g (1 oz) watercress

Juice all the ingredients and serve over ice, decorated with celery sticks, if liked.
Makes 200 ml (7 fl oz)

Nutritional Values

- Kcals 206
- Vitamin C 97 mg
- Potassium 1129 mg
- Magnesium 48 mg

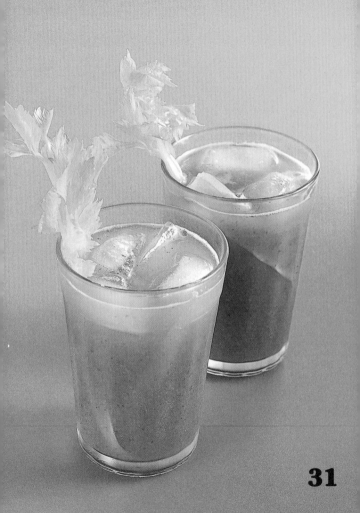

31

This juice is particularly good for the skin, which as the body's largest organ of elimination is the barometer of health and therefore the first to show any imbalances. Encouragingly, the skin is also the first part of the body to show the positive results of detoxifying your system.

herbi-four

175 g (6 oz) red pepper
175 g (6 oz) tomatoes
100 g (3½ oz) white cabbage
1 tablespoon chopped parsley

Juice the red pepper, tomatoes and cabbage. Pour into a tall glass over ice, stir in the parsley and decorate with thin wedges of lime, if liked.
Makes 200 ml (7 fl oz)

Nutritional Values

- Kcals 120
- Vitamin A 4062 iu
- Vitamin C 264 mg
- Selenium 2.13 mcg
- Zinc 1.14 mg

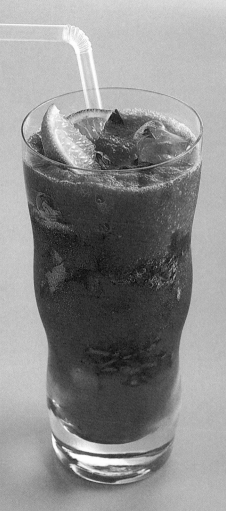

33

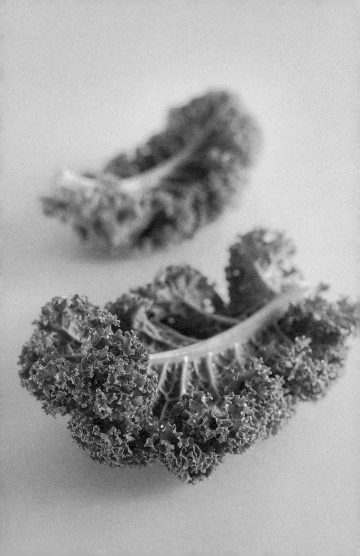

cleanse

A sharp, clean-tasting drink full of vitamins A and C, selenium and zinc, this juice is an excellent internal cleanser.

'c' red

150 g (5 oz) grapefruit
50 g (2 oz) kiwi fruit
175 g (6 oz) pineapple
50 g (2 oz) frozen
    raspberries
50 g (2 oz) frozen
    cranberries

Juice the grapefruit, kiwi fruit and pineapple. Whizz in a blender with the frozen berries. Decorate with raspberries, if liked.

Makes 200 ml (7 fl oz)

Nutritional Values

- Kcals 247
- Vitamin A 693 iu
- Vitamin C 179 mg
- Selenium 4.3 mcg
- Zinc 1.43 mg

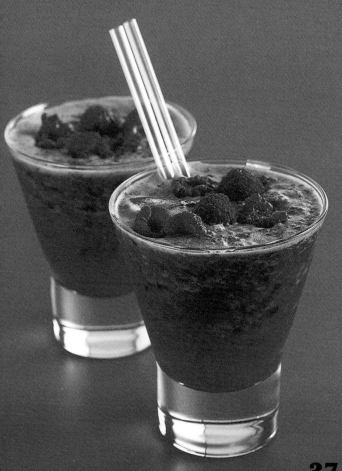

Lettuce and fennel are extremely calming ingredients. They contain calcium and magnesium, which are antispasmodic and produce feelings of calm and wellbeing.

head banger

175 g (6 oz) lettuce
125 g (4 oz) fennel
½ lemon

Juice the lettuce, fennel and lemon, and serve on ice. Decorate with lemon slivers and lettuce leaves, if liked.
Makes 200 ml (7 fl oz)

Nutritional Values

- Kcals 72
- vitamin A 4,726 iu
- vitamin C 67 mg
- potassium 1,070 mg
- calcium 124 mg
- magnesium 32 mg

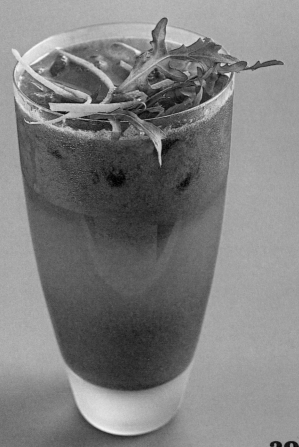

39

This is a particularly good juice to drink after exercise. The cucumber flushes out the kidneys and the grapefruit aids the elimination of toxins.

lemon aid

625 g (1¼ lb) grapefruit flesh
750 g (1½ lb) cucumber
1 lemon, peeled
sparkling mineral water, to top up

Juice the grapefruit, cucumber and lemon. Pour into a jug over ice, and top up with sparkling mineral water. Pour into glasses and decorate with sprigs of mint and slices of lemon, if liked.

Makes 400 ml (14 fl oz)

Nutritional Values

- Kcals 302
- Vitamin C 273 mg
- Potassium 1627 mg
- Magnesium 1332 mg
- Zinc 1.9 mg

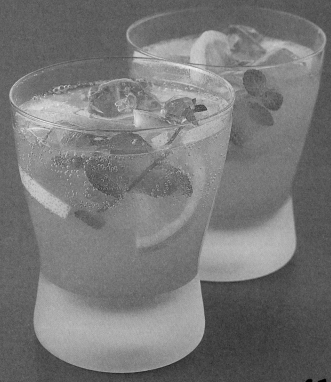

41

Carrot and apple contain pectin, tannic acid and malic acid, which help regulate bowel movement and soothe intestinal walls. Cabbage detoxifies the stomach and upper colon and improves the digestion.

system soother

175 g (6 oz) carrot
250 g (8 oz) apple
125 g (4 oz) red cabbage

Juice all the ingredients, including the apple cores. Serve over ice in a tall glass and decorate with slivers of red cabbage, if liked.
Makes 200 ml (7 fl oz)

Nutritional Values

- Kcals 250
- Vitamin A 49523 iu
- Vitamin C 70 mg
- Potassium 1159 mg
- Selenium 3.79 mcg

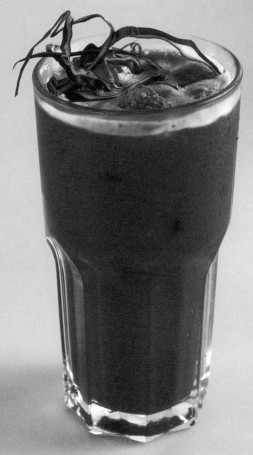

43

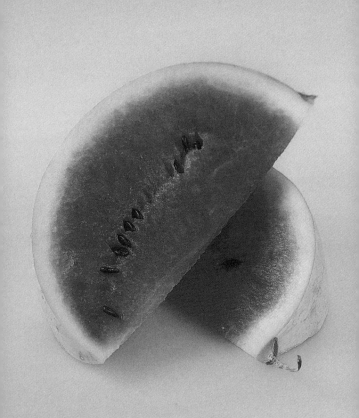

regenerate

Pineapple and grapes are powerful detox fruits and provide a boost of blood sugar, while lettuce and celery both help regenerate the liver and lymph system and aid digestion. All four ingredients can help you sleep.

sleep tight

125 g (4 oz) pineapple
125 g (4 oz) grapes
50 g (2 oz) lettuce
50 g (2 oz) celery

Juice all the ingredients and serve in a tall glass over ice. Decorate with lettuce leaves, if liked.
Makes 200 ml (7 fl oz)

Nutritional Values

- Kcals 167
- Vitamin B6 0.3 mg
- Vitamin C 50 mg
- Magnesium 35.2 mg
- Niacin 1.38 mg
- Tryptophan 4 mg

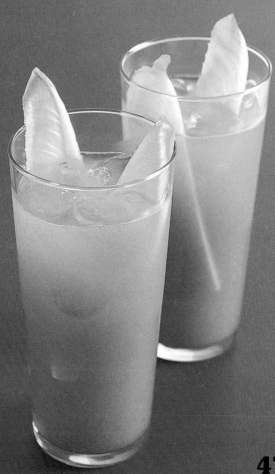

47

The vitamin C and potassium-rich ingredients in this juice help to lower blood pressure.

lounge
lizard

250 g (8 oz) kiwi fruit
125 g (4 oz) cucumber
1 tablespoon
  pomegranate seeds

Wash the kiwi fruit and cucumber but do not peel them, as both contain nutrients in their skins. Juice both and serve with a slice of lime, if liked. If you wish, stir in a tablespoon of pomegranate seeds.
Makes 200 ml (7 fl oz)

Nutritional Values

- Kcals 168
- vitamin C 250 mg
- potassium 1,010 mg
- zinc 0.67 mg

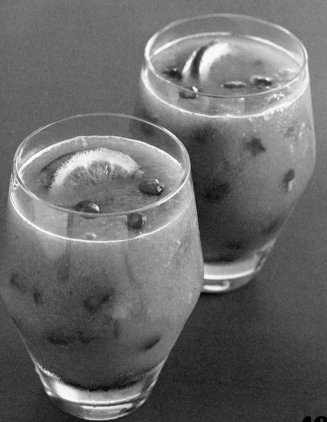

49

A great detoxing and diuretic fruit, watermelon helps speed up the passage of toxin-carrying fluids through the system.

all systems go

¼ watermelon, about
   300 g (10 oz) flesh
2 oranges, peeled

Remove the skin from the watermelon and chop the flesh into even-sized pieces. Juice with the oranges. Pour into a glass and add some ice cubes. Decorate with slices of orange, if liked.
Makes 300 ml (½ pint)

Nutritional Values

- Kcals 200
- Vitamin A 1708 iu
- Vitamin C 170 mg
- Potassium 846 mg
- Iron 1.2 mg
- Calcium 162 mg

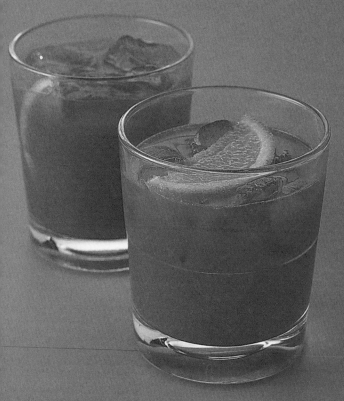

High in fructose, this really flavoursome drink provides instant energy. Pineapple, mango and grapes are fruits with particular detox powers. Both pineapple and mango contain the enzyme bromelin, which helps to produce acids that destroy bad bacteria in the gut, encourage the growth of 'good' bacteria important for digestion, and support tissue repair. Mango also contains the enzyme papain, which helps to break down protein wastes. Grapes help to cleanse the liver and kidneys.

pure cure

100 g (3½ oz) pineapple
100 g (3½ oz) grapes
100 g (3½ oz) orange
 segments
100 g (3½ oz) apple
100 g (3½ oz) mango
 flesh
100 g (3½ oz) peeled
 banana

Juice the pineapple, grapes, orange and apple. Whizz in a blender with the mango, banana and a couple of ice cubes for a super sweet smoothie. Serve decorated with chopped mint and slices of orange, if liked.

Makes 400 ml (14 fl oz)

Nutritional Values

- Kcals 383
- Vitamin A 4631 iu
- Vitamin C 121 mg
- Selenium 3.3 mcg

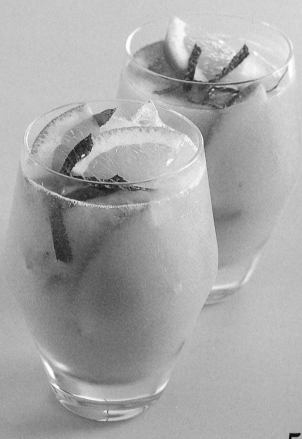

53

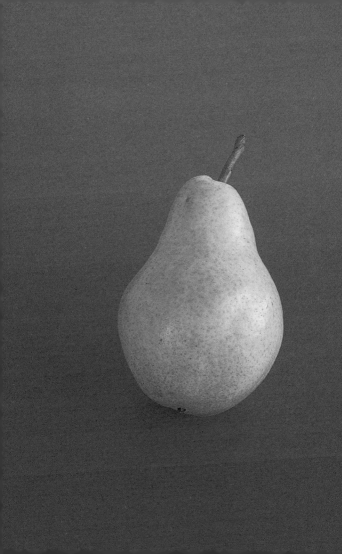

purify

An excellent detoxifier, this juice will prevent the build-up of toxins in your system, which leads to sluggish metabolism, low energy and possibly even serious illnesses. Carrots, lettuce, spinach and celery all work to regenerate the liver and lymph system and aid digestion. Parsley is good for kidney stones, making it the ideal addition to the juice.

squeaky green

175 g (6 oz) carrot
90 g (3 oz) celery
100 g (3½ oz) spinach
100 g (3½ oz) lettuce
25 g (1 oz) parsley

Juice the ingredients and whizz in a blender with a couple of ice cubes. Decorate with sprigs of parsley, if liked.
Makes 200 ml (7 fl oz)

Nutritional Values

- Kcals 137
- Vitamin A 60393 iu
- Vitamin C 120 mg
- Potassium 1855 mg
- Magnesium 138 mg

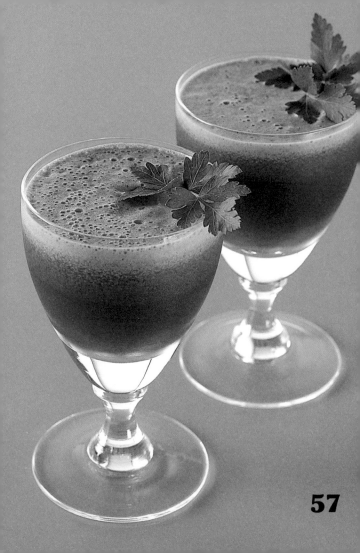

57

Fennel has particularly good detox powers. It also helps to improve digestion and prevent flatulence. Carrots and celery both help the detox process. Available as a powder, spirulina is a form of chlorophyll from the blue-green algae family, which has good energizing properties. In addition, it contains phenylalanine, which suppresses the appetite.

ginger spice

300 g (10 oz) carrot
50 g (2 oz) fennel
75 g (3 oz) celery
2.5 cm (1 inch) cube
   of fresh root ginger,
   roughly chopped
1 tablespoon spirulina
   (optional)

Juice the first four ingredients and serve over ice. Stir in the spirulina, if using. If liked, decorate with strips of fennel and fennel fronds.

Makes 200 ml (7 fl oz)

Nutritional Values

- Kcals 183
- Vitamin A 84600 iu
- Vitamin C 43 mg
- Potassium 1627 mg
- Magnesium 80 mg

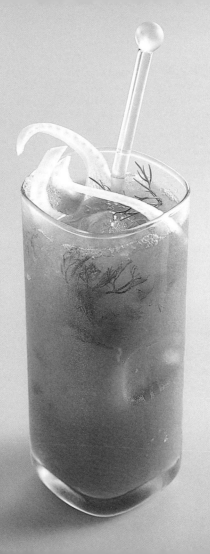

59

This juice contains potassium, phosphorus and chlorine, all of which are good for skin eruptions. Potato juice is not particularly palatable on its own but is an excellent detoxifier. Radishes are also good for detoxification, while the cucumber flushes out the kidneys.

cucumber cleanser

100 g (3½ oz) potato
100 g (3½ oz) radish
100 g (3½ oz) carrot
100 g (3½ oz) cucumber

Juice the ingredients together and whizz in a blender with a couple of ice cubes. Serve in a tumbler over ice decorated with slices of radish, if liked.
Makes 200 ml (7 fl oz)

Nutritional Values

- Kcals 155
- Vitamin C 56 mg
- Potassium 1242 mg
- Phosphorus 128 mg
- Chlorine 920 mg

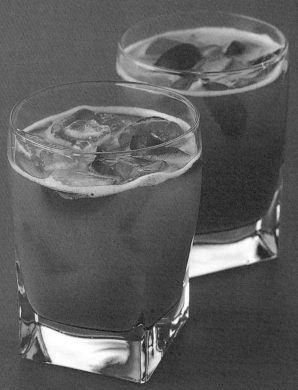

61

Watermelon is the ideal detoxifier, the flesh is packed with beta-carotene and vitamin C. Watermelon juice is so delicious that it's not a chore to drink a glass of this every day. By adding strawberries, you'll be receiving a great boost of vitamin C as well as helping your body fight against bacteria in your system. The juice is also high in zinc and potassium, two great eliminators.

juice boost

200 g (7 oz) watermelon
200 g (7 oz) strawberries

Juice the fruit and whizz in a blender with a couple of ice cubes. Serve decorated with mint sprigs and whole or sliced strawberries, if liked.
Makes 200 ml (7 fl oz)

Nutritional Values

- Kcals 130
- Vitamin A 6562 iu
- Vitamin C 195 mg
- Potassium 950 mg
- Zinc 0.58 mg

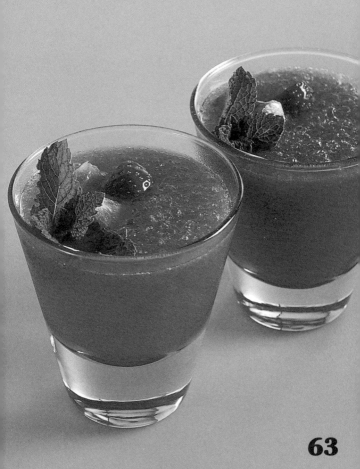

index

acknowledgements

The publisher would like to thank The Juicer Company for the loan of The Champion juicer and the Orange X citrus juicer (featured on pages 12 and 13).

Executive Editor Nicola Hill
Editor Sharon Ashman
Executive Art Editor Geoff Fennell
Designer Sue Michniewicz
Senior Production Controller Jo Sim
Photographer Stephen Conroy
Home Economist David Morgan
Stylist Angela Swaffield
All photographs © Octopus Publishing Group Ltd

ENERGIZE

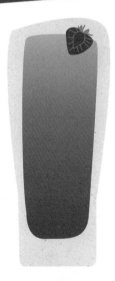

spruce

Safety Note

Energize should not be considered a replacement for professional medical treatment; a physician should be consulted on all matters relating to health. While the advice and information in this book is believed to be accurate, the publisher cannot accept any legal responsibility or liability for any injury or illness sustained while following the advice in this book.

An Hachette UK Company
www.hachette.co.uk

First published in Great Britain in 2017 by Spruce,
a division of Octopus Publishing Group Ltd, Carmelite House,
50 Victoria Embankment, London, EC4Y 0DZ
www.octopusbooks.co.uk
www.octopusbooksusa.com

Distributed in the US by Hachette Book Group,
1290 Avenue of the Americas, 4th and 5th Floors, New York, NY 10104

Distributed in Canada by Canadian Manda Group
664 Annette Street, Toronto, Ontario, Canada M6S 2C8

This material was previously published as *Miracle Juices: Energize*

ISBN 978-1-84601-543-4

A CIP catalogue record for this book is available
from the British Library

Printed and bound in China

10 9 8 7 6 5 4 3 2 1

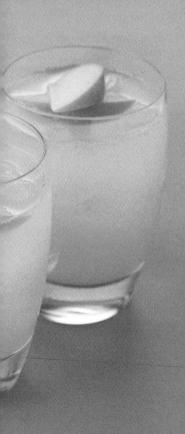

Contents

introduction

Are you always full of energy, bursting to get out there and enjoy every moment life has to offer, or do you often find yourself complaining that you are tired, feeling irritable and lacking enthusiasm? If it is the latter, the answer could lie in the type of food you are eating, because food provides our major source of energy. In order to move, breathe and maintain brain power, we need to consume the right foodstuffs, and many of us undermine this valuable fuel by eating junk food and skipping meals. Add to this a high consumption of alcohol, tea and coffee, sugary drinks, chocolate and smoking and you will be severely limiting your ability to perform at your peak, particularly in times of stress when energy requirements are greater than usual.

Where does our energy come from?

Food is converted into energy during the process of digestion. It is broken down into glucose which is carried to the liver, where it is filtered and stored as glycogen. The pituitary gland in the brain stimulates hormonal releases from the adrenal glands and pancreas, which cause the liver to release the glucose back into the bloodstream when it is needed and it is delivered to whichever organs and muscles require it.

The process of keeping our organs and muscles supplied with the fuel they need is known as blood sugar management. Many different nutrients are required for energy production and a variety of different foods provide the essential blend. Carbohydrates are the key as they are most easily converted into glucose; proteins and fats provide a secondary source of energy, but are equally vital as they provide essential nutrients.

Getting the balance right

The balance between carbohydrates and protein is the lynchpin for sustainable energy and the optimal balance for each person depends on their lifestyle. If you are inactive, elderly or recuperating from an illness, your ratio of protein to carbohydrate should be 1:2. If you lead an active life, then your ideal ratio would be 1:1. Energy requirements are also higher during pregnancy, childhood, puberty and during periods of stress.

glycaemic index

All foods have what is known as a glycaemic index, or GI. This indicates the speed with which they release their sugars into the body. The higher the GI, the quicker the impact on blood sugar levels. Refined foods such as white bread, white rice, sweets and chocolate, commercial cereals and canned drinks all have a high glycaemic value. They will provide an immediate sugar surge, but deplete the body's energy reserves very quickly, leaving a person with less energy than before. It is better to eat foods with a low to moderate GI which supply a constant release of sugar throughout the day.

Low GI foods

- Whole grains (rye, quinoa, millet)
- Soya beans, haricot beans, butter beans, kidney beans
- Chickpeas, lentils
- Yogurt
- Apples, pears, oranges, kiwi fruit, bananas
- Oats
- Wholemeal pasta
- Raw root vegetables

Medium GI foods

- Popcorn
- Sweetcorn
- Potatoes
- Mangoes, apricots, papaya
- Muesli
- Brown rice
- Raisins
- Corn chips

Symptoms of energy imbalance

- Depression
- Irritability
- Mood swings
- Premenstrual tension
- Angry outbursts
- Anxiety and nervousness
- Fatigue
- Lack of concentration
- Continual thirst
- Constant craving for sugar, bread or carbohydrates throughout the day
- Feelings of sluggishness and heaviness in the mornings
- High consumption of stimulants such as tea, coffee, alcohol and carbonated drinks

Boosting energy

Juicing raw vegetables and fruit is a great way to boost energy. Because juices contain no fibre to slow down digestion, the nutrients are readily absorbed and the release of glucose into the bloodstream is rapid. But, to avoid energy peaks and troughs, don't forget to nibble on healthy snacks to help balance blood sugar throughout the day and sustain that vital energy.

The following are good examples.

- Nuts and dried fruit
- Low-fat yogurt with pumpkin seeds and wheatgerm
- Oat and wheatgerm flapjacks
- Crispbread or oatcakes with cheese
- Avocado dip with rice cakes
- Raw vegetables with yogurt or soured cream
- Apple
- Hummus and raw carrot

key nutrients

Nutrient	Function	Sources	Recommended Daily Dosage
Vitamin B1 (thiamine)	Helps convert carbohydrates to glucose; ensures proper oxygenation of the blood for optimal energy release	Brewer's yeast, rice bran, whole grains, raw wheatgerm, green and yellow vegetables, fruit, milk	1.2–1.4 mg (this can be raised to 10–50 mg per day to increase wellbeing)
Vitamin B3 (niacin)	Aids in the metabolism of macronutrients; strengthens digestion; improves blood circulation	Liver, brewer's yeast, raw wheatgerm, fish, eggs, peanuts, dried fruits, avocados	13–18 mg
Vitamin B5 (pantothenic acid)	Stimulates adrenal function; prevents fatigue; reduces stress	Cod roe, meat, raw wheatgerm, whole grains, beans, molasses, nuts, brewer's yeast	10 mg (increase to 30–50 mg when energy is low)
Vitamin B6 (pyridoxine)	Necessary for release of glycogen from the liver when muscles need energy	Brewer's yeast, raw wheatgerm, liver, molasses, cabbage, milk, eggs	1.8–2.2 mg (some nutritionists recommend up to 25 mg)
Vitamin B12 (pyridoxine)	Increases energy; improves brain function; maintains a healthy nervous system	Liver and kidney, meat, eggs, dairy products, spirulina	3 mcg

trient	Function	Sources	Recommended Daily Dosage
lic acid	Necessary for brain function; works as a coenzyme in the breakdown and utilization of proteins	Green leafy vegetables, liver, egg yolk, carrots, cantaloupe melon, pumpkin, avocados, beans	400 mcg
kamin C (corbic d)	Helps to alleviate fatigue, anxiety and depression by assisting in the formation of norepinephrine; used up rapidly by the body during periods of stress	Citrus fruits, peppers, broccoli, tomatoes, cabbage, green leafy vegetables, melons, yams, potatoes	60 mg (many nutritionists recommend 1000–2000 mg to promote immunity, general health and boost energy levels)
agnesium	Helps to balance blood sugar levels and reduce cravings for stimulants; very effective muscle relaxant; vital for energy production of glucose; helps utilize B complex and C vitamins in the body	Figs, lemons, grapefruits, sweetcorn, nuts, apples, raw wheatgerm, green vegetables	350 mg
nc	Involved in carbohydrate metabolism; absorption and action of the B complex vitamins; helps energy production	Raw oysters, meat, fish, raw wheatgerm, mushrooms, pumpkin seeds, egg yolks, dried legumes, milk	15 mg

why juice?

Vital vitamins and minerals such as antioxidants, vitamins A, B, C and E, folic acid, potassium, calcium, magnesium, zinc and amino acids are present in fresh fruits and vegetables, and are all necessary for optimum health. Because juicing removes the indigestible fibre in fruits and vegetables, the nutrients are available to the body in much larger quantities than if the piece of fruit or vegetable were eaten whole. For example, when you eat a raw carrot you are able to assimilate only about 1 per cent of the available beta-carotene, because many of the nutrients are trapped in the fibre. When a carrot is juiced, thereby removing the fibre, nearly 100 per cent of the beta-carotene can be assimilated. Juicing several types of fruits and vegetables on a daily basis is therefore an easy way to ensure that your body receives its full quota of these vital vitamins and minerals.

In addition, fruits and vegetables provide another substance absolutely essential for good health — water.

Most people don't consume enough water. In fact, many of the fluids we drink — coffee, tea, soft drinks, alcoholic beverages and artificially flavoured drinks — contain substances that require extra water for the body to eliminate, and tend to be dehydrating. Fruit and vegetable juices are free of these unnecessary substances.

Your health

A diet high in fruits and vegetables can prevent and help to cure a wide range of ailments. At the cutting edge of nutritional research are the plant chemicals known as phytochemicals, which hold the key to preventing deadly diseases such as cancer and heart disease, and others such as asthma, arthritis and allergies.

Although juicing benefits your overall health and wellbeing, it should be used only to complement your daily eating plan. You must still eat enough from the other food groups (such as grains, dairy food and pulses) to ensure your body maintains strong

bones and healthy cells. If you are
following a specially prescribed diet,
or are under medical
supervision, it is essential
that you discuss any
drastic changes with your
health practitioner before
beginning any type of new
health regime.

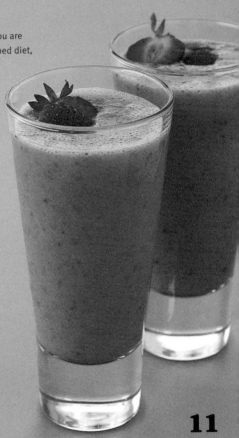

how to juice

Available in a variety of models, juicers work by separating the fruit and vegetable juice from the pulp. Choose a juicer with a reputable brand name, that has an opening big enough for larger fruits and vegetables, and make sure it is easy to take apart and clean, otherwise you may become discouraged from using it.

Types of juicer

A citrus juicer or lemon squeezer is ideal for extracting the juice from oranges, lemons, limes and grapefruit. Pure citrus juice has a high acid content and is best used diluted.

Centrifugal juicers are the most widely used and affordable juicers available. Fresh fruits and vegetables are fed into a rapidly spinning grater, and the pulp separated from the juice by centrifugal force. The pulp is retained in the machine while the juice runs into a separate jug. A centrifugal juicer produces less juice than the more expensive masticating juicer, which works by pulverizing fruits and vegetables, and pushing them through a wire mesh with immense force.

To make smoothies you will need a blender or food processor, as instructed in some recipes.

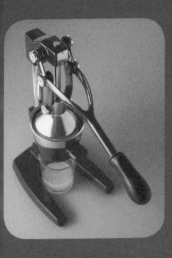

Preparing produce for juicing

It is best to prepare ingredients just before juicing so that fewer nutrients are lost through oxidization. Cut or tear foods into manageable pieces for juicing. If the ingredients are not organic, do not include stems, skins or roots, but if the produce is organic, you can put everything in the juicer. However, don't include the skins from pineapple, mango, papaya, citrus fruit and banana, and remove the stones from avocados, apricots, peaches, mangoes and plums. You can include melon seeds, particularly watermelon, as these are full of juice. For grape juice, choose green grapes with an amber tinge or black grapes with a darkish bloom. Leave the pith on lemons for the pectin content.

Cleaning the juicer

Clean your juicing machine thoroughly, as any residue left may harbour bacterial growth — a toothbrush or nailbrush works well for removing stubborn residual pulp. Leaving the equipment to soak in warm soapy water will loosen the residue from those hard-to-reach places. A solution made up of one part white vinegar to two parts water will lessen any staining produced by the fruits and vegetables.

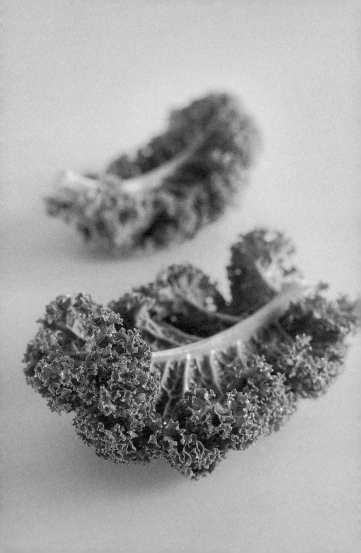

invigorate

Carrots, beetroots and oranges are all high in vitamins A and C, antioxidants and phytonutrients. This juice is also a rich source of potassium. A real tonic which should give your energy levels a boost.

power pack

250 g (8 oz) carrot
125 g (4 oz) beetroot
1 orange
125 g (4 oz) strawberries

Juice the carrot, beetroot and orange. Put the juice into a blender with a couple of ice cubes and the strawberries. Whizz for 20 seconds and serve in a tall glass. Decorate with strips of orange rind, if liked.
Makes 200 ml (7 fl oz)

Nutritional values

- Kcals 244
- Carbohydrate 55 g
- Protein 7 g
- Vitamin C 230 mg
- Vitamin A 2040 IU
- Magnesium 55 mg
- Zinc 1 mg

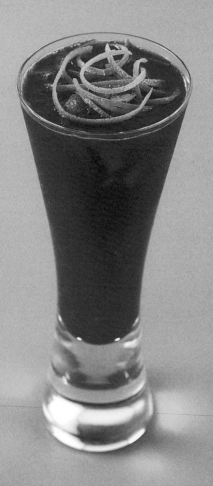

17

Spirulina is one the best sources of vitamin B12, which is essential for the functioning of all cells. Wheatgrass is high in chlorophyll, which combats anaemia. Kale has as much usable calcium as milk. This juice is a great energy booster with nutritional benefits that far outweigh its flavour.

kale and hearty

25 g (1 oz) kale
100 g (3½ oz) wheatgrass
1 teaspoon spirulina

Juice the kale and the wheatgrass, and stir in the spirulina powder. Serve in a small glass decorated with wheatgrass blades.
Makes 50 ml (2 fl oz)

Nutritional values

- Kcals 48
- Carbohydrate 25 g
- Protein 7 g
- Vitamin C 114 mg
- Vitamin A 1186 IU
- Magnesium 64 mg
- Zinc 2 mg

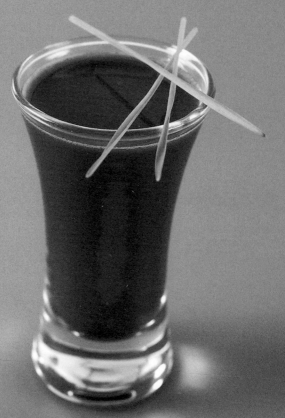

19

High in carbohydrate, this juice is a great energy giver, so it is most suitable after exercise. It can also be a good choice before exercise, however, when high levels of energy will be required. It is also an excellent source of vitamins A and C, potassium, magnesium and phosphorus, and provides useful amounts of iron. To counteract the sweetness of the mango it's best to use a tart variety of apple, such as a Worcester.

energy bubble

3 apples, preferably red
1 mango
2 passion fruit

Wash the apples, peel the mango and remove the stone. Slice the passion fruit in half, scoop out the flesh and discard the seeds. Juice all the ingredients. Pour the juice into a glass and add some ice cubes. Decorate with apple slices, if liked.

Nutritional values

Makes 300 ml (½ pint)

- Kcals 237
- Carbohydrate 58 g
- Protein 3 g
- Vitamin C 80 mg
- Vitamin A 298 IU
- Magnesium 43 mg
- Zinc 1 mg

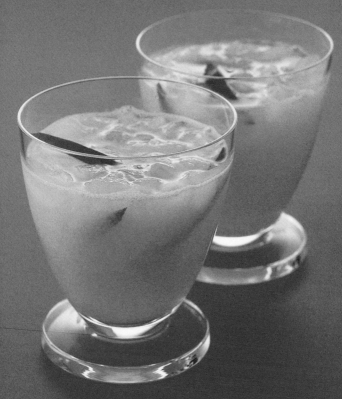

21

This juice contains cinnamon, which is renowned for stabilizing blood sugar. To add a boost of glucose-regulating chromium, stir 1 tablespoon of raw wheatgerm into the finished juice. This juice can help cure hypoglycaemia or very low blood sugar levels which can cause fatigue, light-headedness and depression.

energy burst

125 g (4 oz) spinach
250 g (8 oz) apple
100 g (3½ oz) yellow pepper
pinch of cinnamon

Juice the spinach, apple and pepper, then stir in the cinnamon. Serve in a glass and add a cinnamon stick for decoration, if liked.

Makes 200 ml (7 fl oz)

Nutritional values

- Kcals 175
- Carbohydrate 375 g
- Protein 6 g
- Vitamin C 178 mg
- Vitamin A 466 IU
- Magnesium 98 mg
- Zinc 1 mg

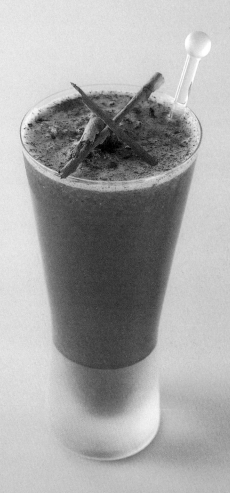

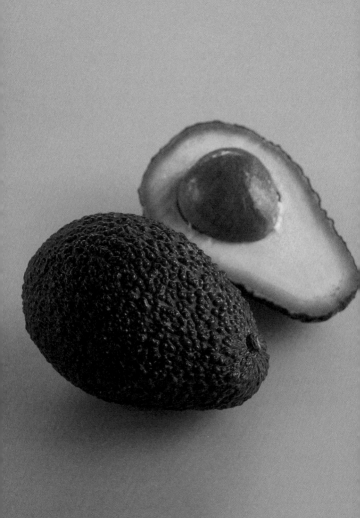

get up
and go

We would run out of paper listing the nutritional aspects of this juice.
Basically it is a great all-round energy booster and the perfect way to perk up
your senses, day or night.

magnificent 7

90 g (3 oz) carrot
50 g (2 oz) green pepper
25 g (1 oz) spinach
25 g (1 oz) onion
50 g (2 oz) celery
90 g (3 oz) cucumber
50 g (2 oz) tomato
sea salt and pepper

Juice all the ingredients and season with
sea salt and pepper. If liked, decorate
with tomato quarters.
Makes 200 ml (7 fl oz)

Nutritional values

• Kcals 75
• Carbohydrate 14 g
• Protein 3 g
• Vitamin C 87 mg
• Vitamin A 872 IU
• Magnesium 35 mg
• Zinc 1 mg

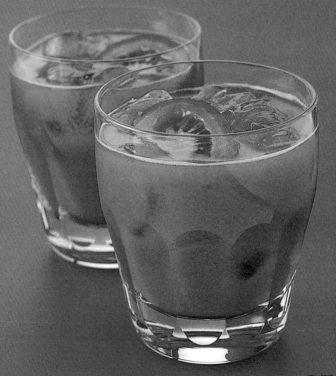

27

A good drink to choose before or after most activities including high-energy sports. Pineapples contain an enzyme, bromelain, that breaks down protein. This juice is rich in B vitamins which help to release energy from carbohydrate. It is an excellent source of vitamins C, B1 and B6, calcium and copper.

sky high

2 pears
½ lime
¼ pineapple, about
   215 g (7½ oz)
   peeled flesh

Juice all the fruit, pour into a glass and add some ice cubes, if wished. Decorate with pieces of pineapple, if liked.
Makes 300 ml (½ pint)

Nutritional values

- Kcals 211
- Carbohydrate 53 g
- Protein 2 g
- Vitamin C 55 mg
- Vitamin A 10 IU
- Magnesium 57 mg
- Zinc 1 mg

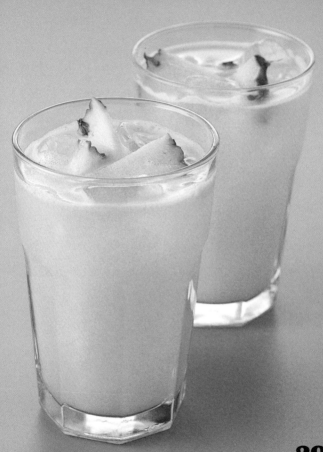

29

High in potassium, vitamin C, vitamin B12 and essential fatty acids, this is a thick shake with a punch. Basically, it is nutritious food, fast. These fruits, in particular the banana, create a feeling of fullness as well as helping to rebalance your sugar levels and thus your energy levels. Your sugar levels will also be helped by the protein in the linseeds. The high levels of vitamin B in the juice will also increase your energy.

high kick

250 g (8 oz) strawberries
125 g (4 oz) kiwi fruit
100 g (3½ oz) banana
1 tablespoon spirulina
1 tablespoon linseeds

Juice the strawberries and kiwi fruit and whizz in a blender with the banana, spirulina, linseeds and a couple of ice cubes. Decorate with redcurrants, if liked.
Makes 200 ml (7 fl oz)

Nutritional values

• Kcals 300
• Carbohydrate 54 g
• Protein 15 g
• Vitamin C 277 mg
• Vitamin A 1503 IU
• Magnesium 132 mg
• Zinc 1 mg

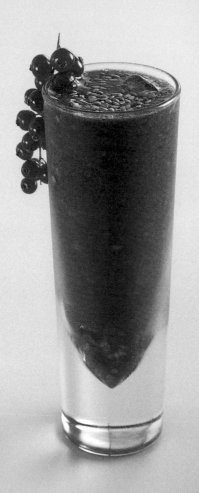

31

This juice provides good amounts of calcium and iron, which make it an excellent energy booster before or during most types of exercise, or just when you need a boost. Calcium is important for good bone health, while the iron helps to prevent fatigue. It is an excellent source of vitamins C, B1 and B2, niacin, B6, folic acid, copper, potassium, calcium, magnesium and phosphorus.

berry bouncer

100 g (3½ oz)
 strawberries
75 g (3 oz) redcurrants
½ orange
125 ml (4 fl oz) water
½ teaspoon clear honey
 (optional)

Hull the strawberries and redcurrants, and peel the orange. Juice the fruit, then add the water. Pour into a glass, stir in the honey, if using, and add some ice cubes. Decorate with redcurrants, if liked.
Makes 250 ml (8 fl oz)

Nutritional values

- Kcals 65
- Carbohydrate 14 g
- Protein 2 g
- Vitamin C 139 mg
- Vitamin A 4 IU
- Magnesium 26 mg
- Zinc 1 mg

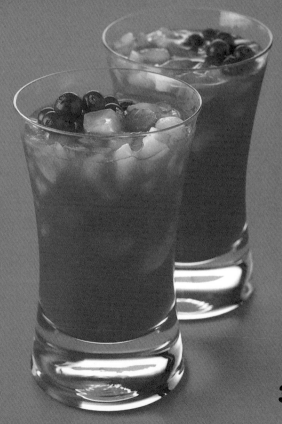

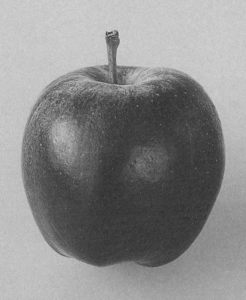

activate

High in water, melons add a refreshing flavour to juices. This juice has quite a high carbohydrate content, so it is good for providing fuel for sports activities. It is an excellent source of vitamins C, B1, B2 and B6, copper, potassium, magnesium and phosphorus and provides useful amounts of calcium. Melon and pineapple are both quite sweet so it's best to use a tart variety of apple such as Granny Smith or Worcester.

liven up

½ **Galia melon, about 400 g (13 oz)**
¼ **pineapple, about 215 g (7½ oz) peeled flesh**
1 **apple**

Remove the skin and seeds from the melon. Juice all the ingredients, pour into a glass and add a couple of ice cubes. Decorate with apple slices, if liked.
Makes 300 ml (½ pint)

Nutritional values

- Kcals 216
- Carbohydrate 52 g
- Protein 3 g
- Vitamin C 90 mg
- Vitamin A 5 IU
- Magnesium 86 mg
- Zinc 1 mg

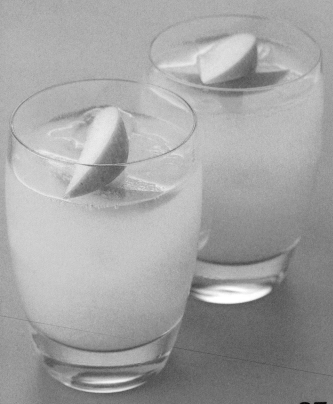

This high-carbohydrate, low-fat smoothie is a great choice for refuelling and soothing tired muscles. Bananas are high in potassium, a vital mineral for muscle and nerve function, which also helps to regulate blood pressure. It is also an excellent source of vitamins C, B1 and B6, folic acid, magnesium and phosphorus.

all nighter

1 small ripe banana
75 g (3 oz) strawberries
250 ml (8 fl oz) orange
   juice

Peel the banana and strawberries. Put the fruit into a freezer container and freeze for at least 2 hours or overnight. Place the frozen fruit and the orange juice in a food processor or blender and process until thick. Decorate with strawberries, if liked, and serve immediately.

Makes 400 ml (14 fl oz)

Nutritional values

- Kcals 180
- Carbohydrate 43 g
- Protein 3 g
- Vitamin C 187 mg
- Vitamin A 7 IU
- Magnesium 65 mg
- Zinc 0.5 mg

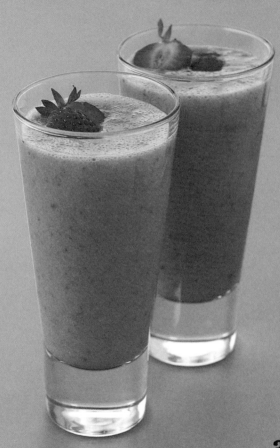

This juice contains large amounts of carbohydrate, essential for refuelling energy stores. The addition of honey gives an extra energy boost. It is an excellent source of vitamins C, B1, B2 and B6, folic acid, calcium, copper and potassium, magnesium and phosphorus.

live wire

2 oranges
1 red apple
1 pear
1 teaspoon clear honey
(optional)

Peel the oranges, juice the flesh with the apple and pear and pour the juice into a glass. Stir in the honey, if using, and add a couple of ice cubes. Decorate with thin orange slices, if liked.
Makes 350 ml (12 fl oz)

Nutritional values

- Kcals 225
- Carbohydrate 54 g
- Protein 4 g
- Vitamin C 188 mg
- Vitamin A 13 IU
- Magnesium 48 mg
- Zinc 1 mg

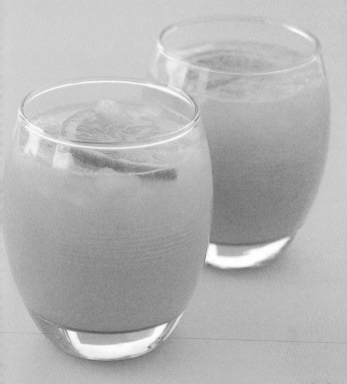

41

Kiwi fruit are an excellent source of vitamin C. This juice will help get you through the day as it contains large amounts of carbohydrate for energy release, plus a hefty amount of vitamin C which may help to increase oxygen uptake and energy production. It is also a good source of vitamins B1 and B6, copper, potassium, magnesium and phosphorus and also provides useful amounts of calcium.

battery charge

2 kiwi fruit
300 g (10 oz) seedless green grapes

Peel the kiwi fruit and juice them with the grapes. Pour the juice into a glass and add a couple of ice cubes. Decorate with kiwifruit slices, if liked.
Makes 300 ml (½ pint)

Nutritional values

- Kcals 239
- Carbohydrate 59 g
- Protein 3 g
- Vitamin C 80 mg
- Vitamin A 10 IU
- Magnesium 39 mg
- Zinc 1 mg

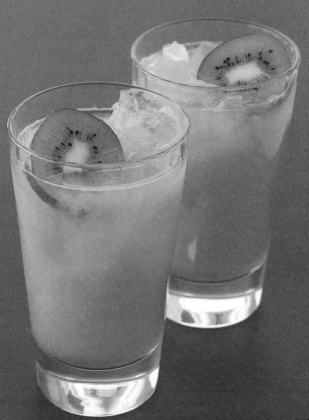

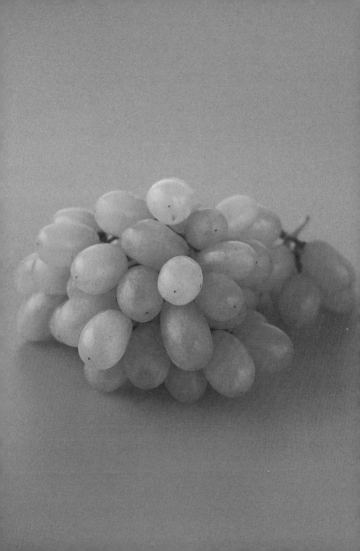

kick start

This isotonic juice is particularly suitable during exercise when a thirst-quenching drink is required. Grapes are a good source of potassium and make the perfect energy snack. This juice is an excellent source of vitamins C, B1 and B6, copper, magnesium and phosphorus.

marathon man

¼ **Galia melon, about 150 g (5 oz)**
75 g (3 oz) seedless green grapes
150 ml (¼ pint) water

Remove the skin and seeds from the melon and juice the fruit. Add the water, pour the juice into a glass and add some ice cubes. Decorate with sliced grapes, if liked.
Makes 300 ml (½ pint)

Nutritional values

- Kcals 87
- Carbohydrate 22 g
- Protein 1 g
- Vitamin C 25 mg
- Vitamin A 1 IU
- Magnesium 24 mg
- Zinc 0.5 mg

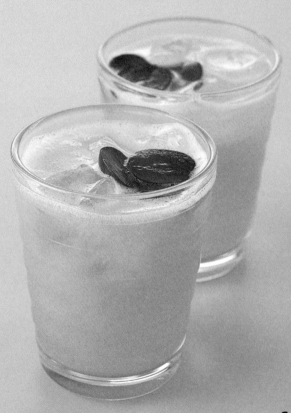

Bananas provide carbohydrate and energy, while avocados supply the body with healthy unsaturated fats. Just one avocado also provides around half the recommended daily intake of vitamin B6. This smoothie is an excellent source of vitamins C, E, B1, B2, B6 and B12, as well as folic acid, calcium, potassium, copper, zinc, magnesium and phosphorus. Drinking this will help to fuel the body and maintain good energy levels. Using skimmed milk helps keep down the overall fat content.

round the clock

1 small ripe avocado
1 small ripe banana
250 ml (8 fl oz) skimmed milk

Peel and stone the avocado, and peel the banana. Place the avocado, banana and milk in a food processor or blender and process until smooth. Pour into a glass, add a couple of ice cubes and drink immediately.

Makes 400 ml (14 fl oz)

Nutritional values

- Kcals 349
- Carbohydrate 33 g
- Protein 11 g
- Vitamin C 17 mg
- Vitamin A 5 IU
- Magnesium 80 mg
- Zinc 2 mg

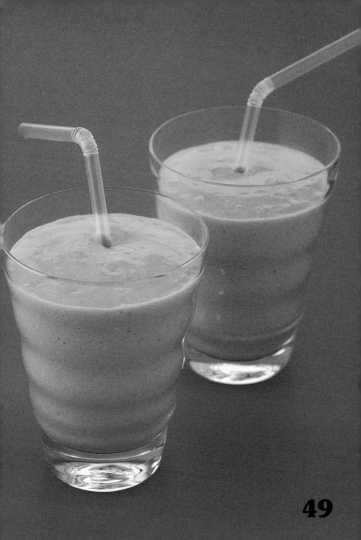

49

This smoothie is a good choice after exercise, when you need a boost. It will help refuel glycogen stores in the muscles and is rich in B vitamins, which help the body to optimize energy production and performance. It is also an excellent source of vitamins A, B1, B2, B6 and C, copper, potassium, magnesium and phosphorus, and provides useful amounts of iron.

rocket fuel

1 ripe mango
300 ml (½ pint) pineapple
juice
rind and juice of ½ lime

Peel and stone the mango, roughly chop the flesh and put it in a freezer container. Freeze for at least 2 hours or overnight. Place the frozen mango in a food processor or blender with the pineapple juice and lime rind and juice and process until thick. Decorate with lime wedges, if liked, and serve immediately.

Nutritional values

Makes 400 ml (14 fl oz)

- Kcals 213
- Carbohydrate 54 g
- Protein 2 g
- Vitamin C 108 mg
- Vitamin A 273 IU
- Magnesium 41 mg
- Zinc 1 mg

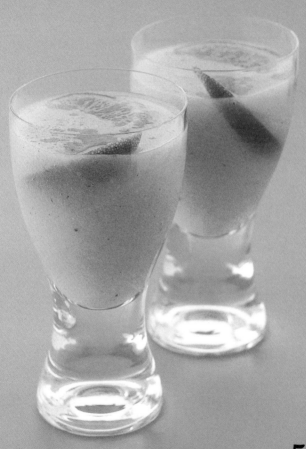

51

The combination of bananas, ground almonds and soya milk makes this a highly nutritious drink. It is best to use very ripe bananas (very yellow skin with black spots) as less ripe ones are largely indigestible. Almonds are an excellent source of vitamin E as well as the minerals calcium, magnesium, phosphorus and copper. They also help to increase the protein content of this drink, which is an excellent source of vitamins C, E, B1, B2 and B6, niacin, folic acid, copper, potassium, zinc, magnesium, phosphorus and provides useful amounts of calcium.

jumping jack

1 very ripe banana
250 ml (8 fl oz) soya milk
20 g (¾ oz) ground
 almonds
pinch of ground cinnamon
a little honey (optional)

Peel and slice the banana, put it into a freezer container and freeze for at least 2 hours or overnight. Place the frozen banana, soya milk, ground almonds and cinnamon in a food processor or blender, add the honey, if using, and process until thick and frothy. Pour into a glass and serve immediately with ice cubes and decorate with ground cinnamon.

Makes 300 ml (½ pint)

Nutritional values

- Kcals 315
- Carbohydrate 47 g
- Protein 9 g
- Vitamin C 11 mg
- Vitamin A 2 IU
- Magnesium 110 mg
- Zinc 1 mg

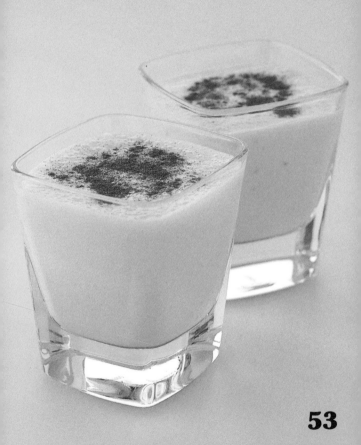

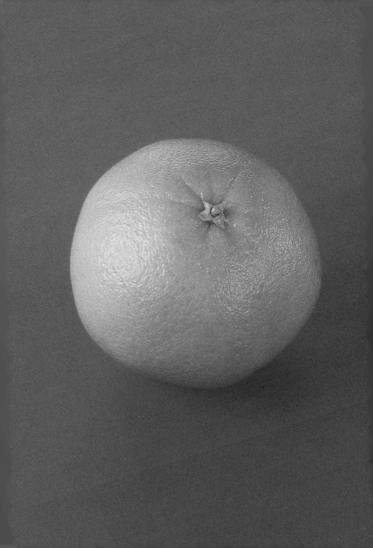

revitalize

Dried apricots have a good concentration of beta-carotene, potassium and iron, making them useful for refuelling muscles and boosting energy levels. Many brands of dried apricots are preserved using sulphur dioxide, which can trigger asthma attacks. To avoid this, check the packaging before you buy, or rinse the apricots well before eating them. This smoothie is an excellent source of vitamins C, B1 and B6, copper, potassium, magnesium and phosphorus and provides useful amounts of calcium and iron.

big boost

65 g (2½ oz) ready-to-eat dried apricots
350 ml (12 fl oz) pineapple juice

Roughly chop the apricots and put them in a large bowl. Pour the pineapple juice over them, cover the bowl and allow to stand overnight. Tip the contents of the bowl into a food processor or blender and process until smooth. Add a couple of ice cubes and drink immediately.
Makes 350 ml (12 fl oz)

Nutritional values

- Kcals 246
- Carbohydrate 61 g
- Protein 4 g
- Vitamin C 39 mg
- Vitamin A 38 IU
- Magnesium 49 mg
- Zinc 1 mg

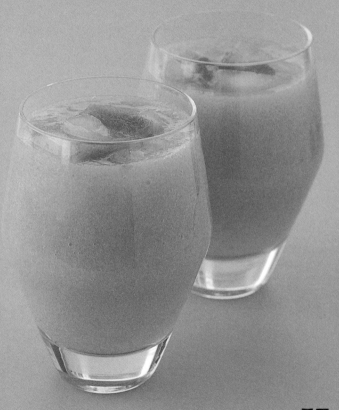

57

Containing high levels of carbohydrate for energy, and calcium for bone health and strength, this smoothie is ideal for people who do a lot of exercise. Cranberry juice is also a natural way to fight urinary tract infections. This smoothie is an excellent source of vitamins A, C, B1, B2, B6 and B12, folic acid, calcium, zinc, potassium, magnesium and phosphorus and also provides useful amounts of iron.

high flyer

1 ripe mango
200 ml (7 fl oz) cranberry
   juice
150 g (5 oz) peach yogurt

Peel and stone the mango and place the flesh in a food processor or blender with the cranberry juice and yogurt and process until smooth. Pour into a glass, add some ice cubes, decorate with cranberries, if liked, and drink immediately.

Makes 400 ml (14 fl oz)

Nutritional values

- Kcals 319
- Carbohydrate 70 g
- Protein 7 g
- Vitamin C 117 mg
- Vitamin A 280 IU
- Magnesium 42 mg
- Zinc 1 mg

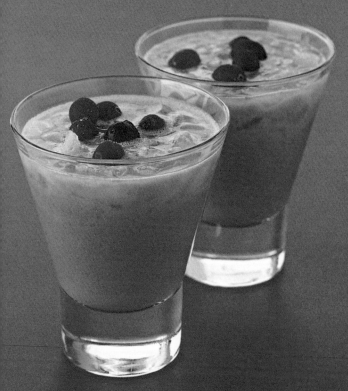

59

As it contains useful amounts of calcium, iron and carbohydrate and has low fat levels, this smoothie replaces energy and raises iron levels, while also helping to maintain bone health. It is an excellent source of vitamins A, C, B1, B2 and B6, folic acid, copper, potassium, magnesium and phosphorus.

quick hit

125 g (4 oz) strawberries
1 small ripe mango
300 ml (½ pint) orange juice

Hull the strawberries, place them in a freezer container and freeze for 2 hours or overnight. Peel and stone the mango, roughly chop the flesh and place it in a food processor or blender with the strawberries and orange juice and process until thick. Decorate with slices of mango, if liked, and serve immediately.

Makes 400 ml (14 fl oz)

Nutritional values

- Kcals 213
- Carbohydrate 52 g
- Protein 4 g
- Vitamin C 290 mg
- Vitamin A 258 IU
- Magnesium 67 mg
- Zinc 0.5 mg

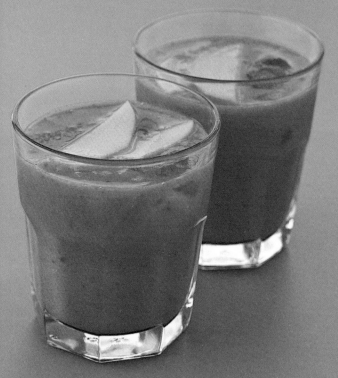

Versatility is the key to this smoothie. It is likely to be well absorbed as it is isotonic, and provides a good energy boost. Adding yogurt to a smoothie is an effective way to increase its content of calcium, which is essential for bone health and strength. Bananas and mangoes supply fibre, making this a filling and satisfying smoothie. It is an excellent source of vitamins A, C, B1, B2 and B6, folic acid, potassium, copper, magnesium and phosphorus.

bionic tonic

1 small banana
½ large ripe mango
75 g (3 oz) natural bio yogurt
150 ml (¼ pint) pineapple juice

Peel and slice the banana then put it in a freezer container and freeze for at least 2 hours or overnight. Peel and stone the mango, roughly chop the flesh and place it in a food processor or blender with the frozen banana, yogurt and pineapple juice. Process until smooth and serve immediately, decorated with pineapple chunks, if liked.

Makes 300 ml (½ pint)

Nutritional values

- Kcals 240
- Carbohydrate 50 g
- Protein 6 g
- Vitamin C 56 mg
- Vitamin A 161 IU
- Magnesium 60 mg
- Zinc 1 mg

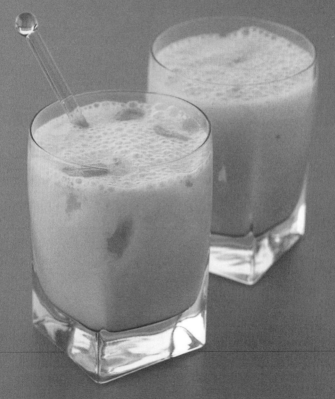

index

acknowledgements

The publisher would like to thank The Juicer Company
for the loan of The Champion juicer and the Orange X
citrus juicer (featured on pages 12 and 13).

Executive Editor Nicola Hill
Editor Abi Rowsell
Executive Art Editor Geoff Fennell
Designer Sue Michniewicz
Senior Production Controller Jo Sim
Photographer Stephen Conroy
Home Economist David Morgan
Stylist Angela Swaffield
All photographs © Octopus
Publishing Group Ltd

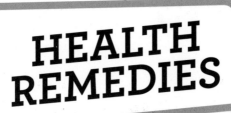

HEALTH REMEDIES

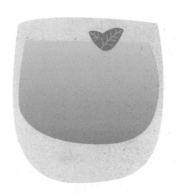

spruce

An Hachette UK Company
www.hachette.co.uk

First published in Great Britain in 2017 by Spruce,
a division of Octopus Publishing Group Ltd, Carmelite House,
50 Victoria Embankment, London, EC4Y 0DZ
www.octopusbooks.co.uk
www.octopusbooksusa.com

Copyright © Octopus Publishing Group Ltd 2017

Distributed in the US by Hachette Book Group,
1290 Avenue of the Americas, 4th and 5th Floors, New York, NY 10104

Distributed in Canada by Canadian Manda Group
664 Annette Street, Toronto, Ontario, Canada M6S 2C8

This material was previously published as *Miracle Juices: Health
Remedies*

ISBN 978-1-84601-543-4

A CIP catalogue record for this book is available
from the British Library

Printed and bound in China

10 9 8 7 6 5 4 3 2 1

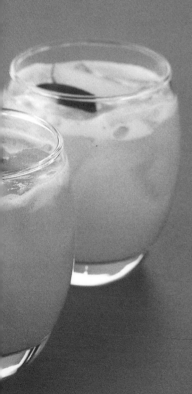

Contents

introduction

It would be a wonderful world if we were all fit and healthy, and free from disease, but unfortunately this just isn't the case. All too often our hectic lifestyles mean that we are stressed out, living and working in polluted environments, not exercising regularly and relying on stimulants such as tea, coffee, alcohol and cigarettes.

Even though we know we should be eating healthily and having at least five portions of fresh fruit and vegetables a day, the sad truth is very different. Many of us eat junk food and think sitting down to an evening meal means piercing the plastic film on a dish of processed food before popping it in the microwave.

It is no wonder that many people spend their time feeling tired and irritable, have trouble sleeping and always seem to be fighting off colds or other minor infections. This leads us to the doctor for painkillers and antibiotics, which may clear up the symptoms, but do not deal with the cause. In fact, regular courses of antibiotics upset the natural balance of our bodies by destroying not only the unwanted bacteria that are causing the infection, but also the beneficial bacteria in our digestive system as well. This can create another set of unpleasant symptoms. Read the list of possible side effects on any packet of prescribed drugs, they all tell the same story. It becomes a vicious circle, where our bodies are the ultimate losers.

Living like this over a prolonged period of time may weaken our immune systems to such an extent that it predisposes us to chronic degenerative diseases later in life.

By eating a balanced diet of fresh and, preferably, organic, food, we can strengthen our bodies and feel energized and healthy. If you are suffering from certain ailments, or determined to prevent further disease, there are many combinations of fruit and vegetables that can help if combined with a healthy eating plan that includes nutritious ingredients from the other vital food groups, such as proteins and fats.

So what makes fresh fruit and vegetables miracle remedies?

They are packed full of antioxidants, vitamins, minerals and enzymes that haven't been destroyed by processing and packing. Once fruits and vegetables have been juiced, the body assimilates their nutrients very rapidly. This can make them potent tonics. The juice is also a valuable source of water, which is essential to good health, particularly as many of the fluids we do drink deplete the body of vital water. Tea, coffee, alcohol, soft drinks and artificially flavoured drinks are all dehydrating to the system.

For those people who don't eat the recommended minimum five portions of fruit and vegetables a day, a juice will go a long way towards providing the body with those vital nutrients.

The juices in this book are aimed at certain conditions and will alleviate symptoms, and, if taken regularly, they will act as preventative agents in the fight against ill health. But they can't do it on their own.

In order to give yourself the best possible chance of remaining fit and full of vigour, you have to give it one hundred percent. Cut down on alcohol, junk food, tea, coffee and fizzy drinks, and give up cigarettes. Exercise regularly and eat nutritious food. Your body will love you for it.

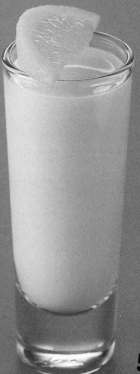

common conditions

Condition	Juices that can help	Harmful influences
Anaemia	Iron Maiden, Heart Beet	Insecticides, excessive use of laxatives, tea and coffee (interfere with iron absorption)
Arthritis	Twister	Fatty foods, refined carbohydrates, excessive alcohol, food allergies
Bloating	Fine and Dandy, Bumpy Ride	Salty food, food allergies
Cellulite	Bumpy Ride, Fine and Dandy	Alcohol, smoking, junk food, lack of exercise
High cholesterol	Purple Passion, Heart Beet, Belly Berry	Saturated fats, stress, cigarettes, refined carbohydrates
Constipation	Way to Go, Healing Hand	Prolonged use of chemical laxatives, fatigue, stress, poor diet, lack of fluids
Diarrhoea	Belly Berry, Purple Passion	Bacterial infection from food poisoning, stress, antibiotics, dairy intolerance, alcohol
Eyesight	Twister, Vision Impeccable	Computers, fatigue, allergies, lack of A, C and E vitamins
Low fertility	Heart Beet, Earth Mother, Passion Thriller, Cool Down	Stress, poor diet, alcohol, smoking, caffeine

Condition	Juices that can help	Harmful influences
Heart disease	Heart Beet, Bumpy Ride, Purple Passion	Heavy meals, refined starches, hydrogenated and saturated fats, sugar
Menopause	Cool Down, Heart Beet	Refined food, alcohol
Motion sickness	Quantum Leap	Fatty foods, alcohol, stress, certain drugs
Muscle damage	Healing Hand	Stress, lack of potassium and magnesium, diuretics, lack of protein
Osteoporosis	Sticks and Stones	Alcohol, salty foods, coffee, carbonated drinks, smoking
Pregnancy	Earth Mother, Cool Down	Alcohol, nutritional deficiencies (especially folic acid)
Pre-menstrual tension	Berry Booster, Fine and Dandy, Bumpy Ride	Stress, junk food, alcohol, caffeine
Sinusitis	Loosen Up 1, Loosen Up 2	Smoking, alcohol, allergies, dairy foods
Stomach ulcer	Well Healed	Painkillers, poor diet, fatty food, coffee, smoking, alcohol, fizzy drinks
Thrush	Live and Kicking, Belly Berry	Coffee, antibiotics, sugar

top five fruits

Fruit	Nutrients	Benefits
Strawberries	Vitamins A, C and K, beta-carotene, folic acid, potassium	Anti-cancer, anti-viral, anti-bacterial
Apple	Vitamin C, calcium, magnesium, phosphorus, beta-carotene, pectin	Astringent, tonic, relieves constipation, reactivates beneficial gut bacteria, reduces cholesterol, helps remove toxins
Kiwi fruit	Vitamin C, magnesium, phosphorus, potassium	Removes excess sodium in the body, excellent source of digestive enzymes
Orange	Vitamin C, calcium, potassium, beta-carotene, folic acid	Cleansing, internal antiseptic, stimulates peristalsis
Banana	Vitamins B6, C and K, potassium, tryptophan, beta-carotene	Promotes sleep, mild laxative, anti-fungal, natural antibiotic, helps ulcers, lowers cholesterol, helps to remove toxic metals from the body

top five vegetables

Vegetable	Nutrients	Benefits
Broccoli	Vitamins C, B3 and B5, calcium, magnesium, phosphorus, beta-carotene, folic acid	Anti-cancer, antioxidant, intestinal cleanser, excellent source of fibre, antibiotic, anti-viral, stimulates liver
Carrot	Calcium, magnesium, potassium, phosphorus, beta-carotene	Excellent detoxifier and food for the liver and digestive tract, helps kidney function, anti-viral, anti-bacterial
Cabbage	Vitamins C, E and K, calcium, magnesium, potassium, phosphorus, beta-carotene, folic acid, iodine	Eaten raw, it detoxifies the stomach and the upper colon, improves digestion, stimulates the immune system, kills bacteria and viruses. Anti-cancer, antioxidant
Beetroot	Vitamin C, calcium, magnesium, iron, phosphorus, potassium, manganese, folic acid	Good intestinal cleanser, eliminates kidney stones, blood builder, detoxifies liver and gall bladder
Tomato	Vitamin C, calcium, magnesium, phosphorus, beta-carotene, folic acid	Hydrating, antiseptic, alkaline, reduces liver inflammation, and contains lycopene which is an effective anti-cancer agent

why juice?

Vital vitamins and minerals such as antioxidants, vitamins A, B, C and E, folic acid, potassium, calcium, magnesium, zinc and amino acids are present in fresh fruits and vegetables, and are all necessary for optimum health. Because juicing removes the indigestible fibre in fruits and vegetables, the nutrients are available to the body in much larger quantities than if the piece of fruit or vegetable were eaten whole. For example, when you eat a raw carrot you are able to assimilate only about 1 per cent of the available beta-carotene because many of the nutrients are trapped in the fibre. When a carrot is juiced, thereby removing the fibre, nearly 100 per cent of the beta-carotene can be assimilated. Juicing several types of fruits and vegetables on a daily basis is therefore an easy way to ensure that your body receives its full quota of these vital vitamins and minerals.

In addition, fruits and vegetables provide another substance absolutely essential for good health — water.

Most people don't consume enough water. In fact, many of the fluids we drink — coffee, tea, soft drinks, alcoholic beverages and artificially flavoured drinks — contain substances that require extra water for the body to eliminate, and tend to be dehydrating. Fruit and vegetable juices are free of these unnecessary substances.

Your health

A diet high in fruits and vegetables can prevent and help to cure a wide range of ailments. At the cutting edge of nutritional research are the plant chemicals known as phytochemicals, which hold the key to preventing deadly diseases such as cancer and heart disease, and others such as asthma, arthritis and allergies.

Although juicing benefits your overall health, it should be used only to complement your daily eating plan. You must still eat enough from the other food groups (such as grains, dairy food and pulses) to ensure your body maintains strong bones and

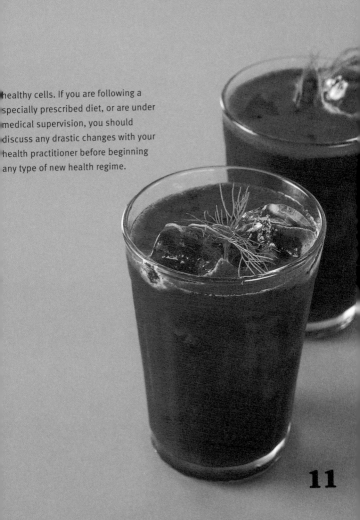

healthy cells. If you are following a specially prescribed diet, or are under medical supervision, you should discuss any drastic changes with your health practitioner before beginning any type of new health regime.

11

how to juice

Available in a variety of models, juicers work by separating the fruit and vegetable juice from the pulp. Choose a juicer with a reputable brand name, that has an opening big enough for larger fruits and vegetables, and make sure it is easy to take apart and clean, otherwise you may become discouraged from using it.

Types of juicer

A citrus juicer or lemon squeezer is ideal for extracting the juice from oranges, lemons, limes and grapefruit, especially if you want to add just a small amount of citrus juice to another liquid. Pure citrus juice has a high acid content, which may upset your stomach, so it is best diluted.

Centrifugal juicers are the most widely used and affordable juicers available. Fresh fruits and vegetables are fed into a rapidly spinning grater, and the pulp separated from the juice by centrifugal force. The pulp is retained in the machine while the juice runs into a separate jug. A centrifugal juicer produces less juice than the more expensive masticating juicer, which works by pulverizing fruits and vegetables, and pushing them through a wire mesh with immense force.

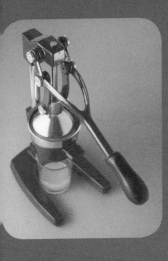

Preparing produce for juicing

It is best to prepare ingredients just before juicing so that fewer nutrients are lost through oxidization. Cut or tear foods into manageable pieces for juicing. If the ingredients are not organic, do not include stems, skins or roots, but if the produce is organic, you can put everything in the juicer. However, don't include the skins from pineapple, mango, papaya, citrus fruit and banana, and remove the stones from avocados, apricots, peaches, mangoes and plums. You can include melon seeds, particularly watermelon, as these are full of juice. For grape juice, choose green grapes with an amber tinge or black grapes with a darkish bloom. Leave the pith on lemons for the pectin content.

Cleaning the juicer

Clean your juicing machine thoroughly, as any residue left may harbour bacterial growth — a toothbrush or nailbrush works well for removing stubborn residual pulp. Leaving the equipment to soak in warm soapy water will loosen the residue from those hard-to-reach places. A solution made up of one part white vinegar to two parts water will lessen any staining produced by the fruits and vegetables.

13

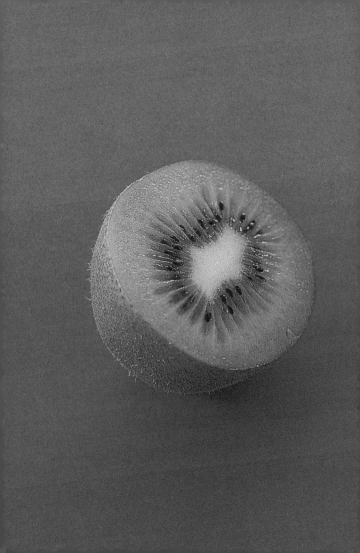

zest

THRUSH. Candida albicans is a common yeast which lives harmlessly in all of us. However, in some cases of low immunity, it can travel through the vaginal tract and cause thrush. Symptoms include mood swings and depression, recurrent vaginal yeast and chronic digestive problems. Cut out junk food, fats, sugar and highly processed foods to discourage the growth of yeast. All the ingredients in this juice have antibacterial properties. It is particularly effective if you are taking antibiotics.

live and kicking

250 g (8 oz) apple
100 g (3½ oz) frozen cranberries
100 g (3½ oz) live natural yogurt
1 tablespoon clear honey

Juice the apple and whizz in a blender with the other ingredients. Serve in a tumbler over ice cubes.
Makes 200 ml (7 fl oz)

Nutritional values

- Kcals 339
- Vitamin C 20 mg
- Calcium 40 mg

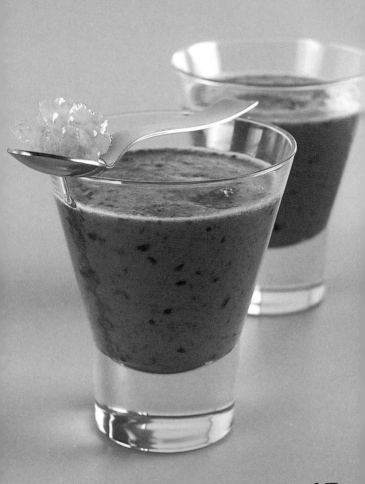

17

LOW FERTILITY. With low sperm counts and lowered fertility levels, our reproductive abilities are one of the biggest causes of concern in today's society. Male fertility may be boosted by increasing intakes of vitamin E, zinc and iron. Women should look to increase their folic acid levels, as well as zinc and vitamin E. Avocado is rich in vitamin E, while apricots are an excellent source of zinc and iron.

passion thriller

175 g (6 oz) melon
  (½ large melon)
125 g (4 oz) cucumber
125 g (4 oz) avocado
50 g (2 oz) dried apricots
1 tablespoon wheatgerm

Juice the melon and cucumber. Whizz in a blender with the avocado, apricots, wheatgerm and a couple of ice cubes. Decorate with dried apricot slivers, if liked.

Makes 200 ml (7 fl oz)

Nutritional values

- Kcals 357
- Vitamin A 8,738 iu
- Vitamin C 110 mg
- Vitamin E 2 mcg
- Potassium 1,470 mg
- Iron 1.6 mg
- Zinc 1.29 mg

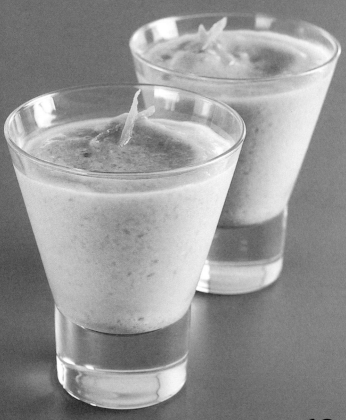

PMS. If you are one of the many women who suffer from monthly cramps, irritability and stomach upsets due to your menstrual cycle, then help is at hand! It is important to ensure that you are replacing your iron levels, as many women find that they are lethargic and tired during their period. If you also feel bloated due to water retention, or find that you gain weight just before your period, then certain fruits and vegetables may assist these symptoms. Your cycle may also affect your moods, so a calming juice may be just what you need to ensure that your cycle causes as little disruption as possible. Pineapples contain bromelain which is a great muscle relaxant, and blackberries are good sources of folic acid.

berry booster

375 g (12 oz)
   blackberries
375 g (12 oz) pineapple
   or 1 small pineapple

Juice the blackberries first, then the pineapple, to push through the pulp. Blend the juice with a couple of ice cubes and serve in a tall glass, decorated with a pineapple sliver, if liked.
Makes 200 ml (7 fl oz)

Nutritional values

- Kcals 353
- Vitamin A 658 iu
- Vitamin C 129.5 mg
- Iron 3.29 mg
- Potassium 1,081 mg
- Calcium 136 mg
- Folic acid 340 mcg

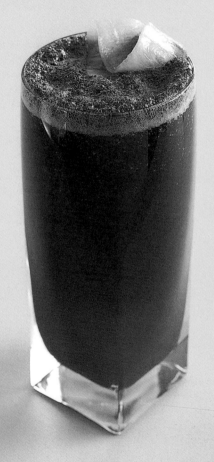

21

MENOPAUSE. The menopause occurs when the amount of the hormones oestrogen and progesterone produced by the ovaries decreases. This can be an extremely stressful time for women, as the menopause may cause irritability, hot flushes, mood swings, headaches, night sweats, vaginal dryness, loss of libido and anxiety. Beetroot is a rich source of folate which can help to protect the heart, and, together with carrots, helps to regulate hormones. Yam provides the hormone progesterone, which helps to replace the hormones lost when the menopause occurs.

cool down

175 g (6 oz) carrot
100 g (3½ oz) beetroot
175 g (6 oz) yam or
    sweet potato
125 g (4 oz) fennel

Juice all the ingredients. Mix well and serve in a glass with ice cubes. Decorate with fennel fronds, if liked.
Makes 200 ml (7 fl oz)

Nutritional values

- Kcals 296
- Vitamin A 49,430 iu
- Vitamin C 69.95 mg
- Iron 3.9 mg
- Folic acid 254 mcg
- Folate 196 mcg

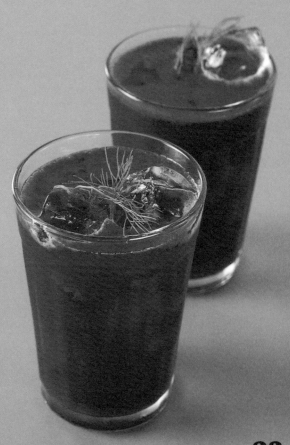

23

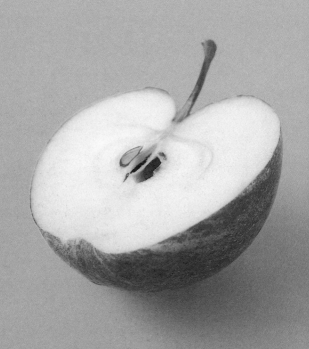

tonic

CELLULITE. The lumpy orange-peel skin that afflicts even the slimmest of women has baffled scientists and medical professionals for years. It is caused by the immobilization of fat cells, and if we eat a diet which is low in the saturated fats found in meat and dairy products this will ensure that fat cells disperse. Large amounts of water to flush out toxins, as well as fruits and vegetables with a high water content, all help to eliminate cellulite.This juice cleanses the whole system – blood, kidneys and lymph. The pectin in the apples strengthens the immune system.

bumpy ride

200 g (7 oz) apple
50 g (2 oz) beetroot
90 g (3 oz) celery

Juice together all the ingredients and serve over ice in a tumbler. Decorate with apple slices, if liked.
Makes 150 ml (¼ pint)

Nutritional values

- Kcals 179
- Vitamin A 480 iu
- Vitamin C 23 mg
- Potassium 763 mg
- Magnesium 37 mg

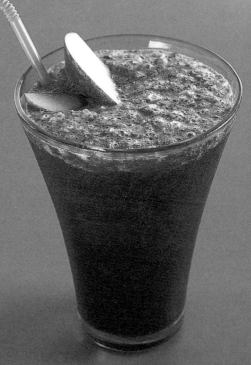

27

SINUSITIS. Sinus problems occur when the nasal and sinus passages become inflamed. Keep away from smoky places and try to avoid exhaust fumes, dust and pollen. Dairy products and wheat are also mucus-forming, so cut these out of your diet, if you can, until your condition has improved. Loosen Up 1 and Loosen Up 2 on the next page should be taken in tandem. Horseradish stimulates capillary action and dissolves mucus in the nasal passages, while the vitamin C in lemon juice may help to lower a high temperature.

loosen up 1

1½ teaspoons pulverized horseradish
½ lemon

Pulverize the horseradish by juicing a small amount and mixing the juice and the pulp. Put it into a shot glass and stir in the lemon juice. Take twice a day. **Makes 50 ml (2 fl oz)**

Nutritional values

- Kcals 25
- Vitamin C 55 mg
- Selenium 0.4 mcg
- Zinc 0.18 mg

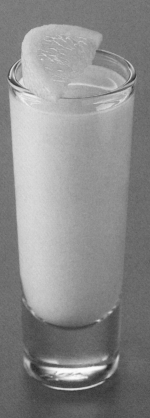

29

SINUSITIS. This juice should be taken one hour after Loosen Up 1 on page 30. The radish juice is too strong to be taken alone, but combined with carrot it has the effect of soothing the membranes and cleansing the body of the mucus dissolved by the horseradish in Loosen Up 1.

loosen up 2

175 g (6 oz) carrot
100 g (3½ oz) radishes,
 with tops and leaves
2.5 cm (1 inch) cube
 fresh root ginger,
 roughly chopped
 (optional)

Juice the carrot, radishes and ginger, if using. Add some ice cubes. Drink one hour after Loosen Up 1.
Makes 200 ml (7 fl oz)

Nutritional values

- Kcals 115
- Vitamin A 49,233 iu
- Vitamin C 40 mg
- Selenium 2.82 mcg
- Zinc 0.8 mg

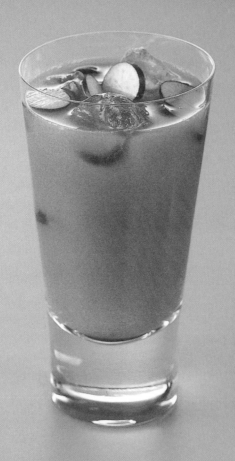

31

BLOATING OR WATER RETENTION. This can be uncomfortable and painful. The problem can be caused by food allergies, hormonal imbalances, a lack of essential fatty acids in the diet, and also, ironically, by not drinking enough water. All the ingredients in this juice contain high levels of zinc and potassium. This recipe is also great if you have just eaten a salty meal. Zinc is essential to decrease water retention.

fine and dandy

125 g (4 oz) asparagus
   spears
10 dandelion leaves
125 g (4 oz) melon
175 g (6 oz) cucumber
200 g (7 oz) pear

Trim the woody bits off the asparagus spears. Roll the dandelion leaves into a ball and juice them (if you have picked wild leaves, wash them first) with the asparagus. Peel and juice the melon. Juice the cucumber and pear with their skins. Whizz everything in a blender and serve in a tall glass with ice cubes.

Makes 200 ml (7 fl oz)

Nutritional values

• Kcals 215
• Vitamin A 5,018 iu
• Vitamin C 87 mg
• Potassium 1,235 mg
• Zinc 1.36 mg

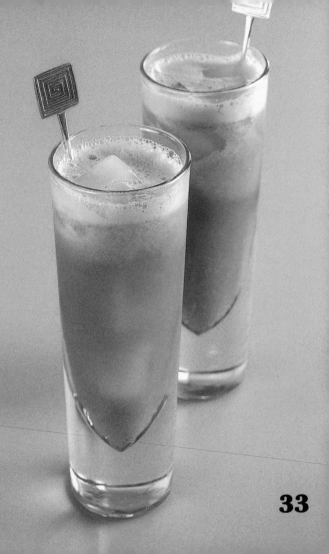

33

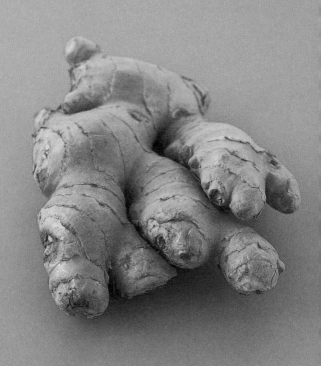

wellbeing

HEART DISEASE. This is one of the most preventable diseases in today's society. An increased intake of fried and fatty foods, a high salt intake, stress, smoking and lack of exercise are all contributory factors. Boosting your intake of vitamin C and vitamin E and taking regular exercise can add as many as ten years to your life. The onion and garlic thin the blood and help to lower cholesterol. Watercress oxygenates the blood and beetroot builds up the red blood cells.

heart beet

125 g (4 oz) beetroot
125 g (4 oz) watercress
125 g (4 oz) red onion
250 g (8 oz) carrot
1 garlic clove

Juice the ingredients and serve in a tall glass. Decorate with beet leaves and watercress, if liked.

Makes 200 ml (7 fl oz)

Nutritional values

- Kcals 167
- Vitamin A 41,166 iu
- Vitamin C 85 mg
- Magnesium 85 mg
- Niacin 2 mg
- Vitamin B6 0.56 mg
- Vitamin E 2.36 mg

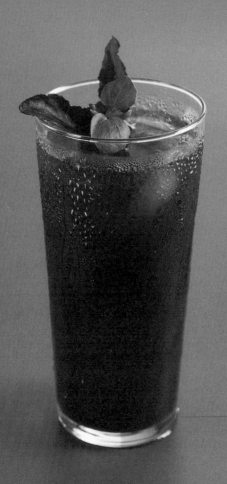

REDUCING CHOLESTEROL. High cholesterol levels are caused by eating a diet containing too much saturated fat, which leads to a build-up along the inside walls of the arteries. Grapefruit is particularly recommended for its rich source of vitamin C and bioflavonoids, which protect the health of the arteries. Blueberries are also extremely potent antioxidants and, along with apples, can help prevent hardening of the arteries and reduce cholesterol levels.

purple passion

250 g (8 oz) blueberries
125 g (4 oz) grapefruit
250 g (8 oz) apple
2.5 cm (1 inch) cube
fresh root ginger,
roughly chopped

Juice all the ingredients and serve in a tall glass with ice cubes. Decorate with thin slices of ginger, if liked.
Makes 200 ml (7 fl oz)

Nutritional values

- Kcals 380
- Vitamin A 695 iu
- Vitamin C 134 mg
- Magnesium 59 mg
- Niacin 1.91 mg
- Vitamin B6 0.39 mg
- Vitamin E 3.12 mg

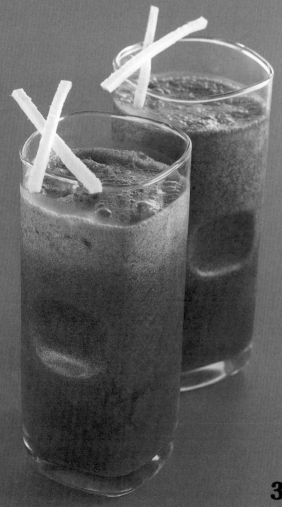

ANAEMIA. If you lack iron in your diet (possibly due to a vegetarian diet, or a heavy menstrual cycle) then you may have anaemia, which can leave you feeling lethargic, depressed, or prone to flu and colds. Folic acid builds up red blood cells, chlorophyll helps to combat fatigue, and spirulina provides a valuable boost of vitamin B12.

iron maiden

250 g (8 oz) spinach
25 g (1 oz) parsley
250 g (8 oz) carrot
1 teaspoon spirulina

Juice the spinach, parsley and carrot and stir in the spirulina. Serve in a tumbler, decorated with carrot slivers, if liked.
Makes 200 ml (7 fl oz)

Nutritional values

- Kcals 229
- Vitamin C 450 mg
- Folic acid 235 mg
- Chlorophyll 100 mg
- Vitamin B12 20 mcg

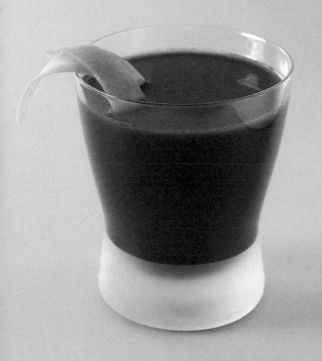

41

MOTION SICKNESS. If even the thought of travelling by boat or plane, or by any form of transport which has a constant rocking motion, makes you feel queasy then a fresh ginger juice may provide the solution. (One teaspoon of dried ginger in apple juice works well, if you are on the move.) Said to be more effective than anything else you can buy over the counter, ginger is ideal for quelling nausea. Drink just before travelling.

quantum
leap

250 g (8 oz) apple
2.5 cm (1 inch) cube
**   fresh root ginger,**
**   roughly chopped**

Juice the apple and ginger and serve in a glass over ice. Decorate with apple slices, if liked. This drink can be diluted with sparkling mineral water to taste.
Makes 100 ml (3½ fl oz)

Nutritional values

- Kcals 160
- Vitamin C 16 mg

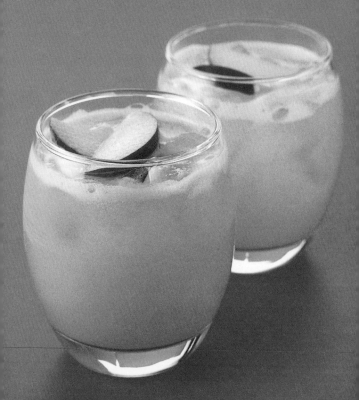

43

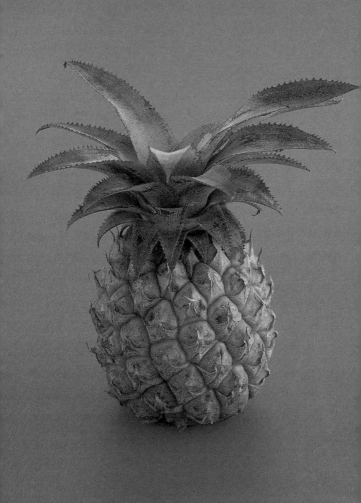

vitality

STOMACH ULCERS. These are caused by excess acid and the digestive enzyme pepsin and are aggravated by stress, smoking and acidic food and drinks. They can be controlled by keeping your intake as alkaline as possible, but if you have severe abdominal pain you must always consult a doctor. Both carrot and cabbage juices are renowned for having a healing effect on stomach ulcers.

well healed

250 g (8 oz) carrot
250 g (8 oz) green
   cabbage

Juice the vegetables and serve in a tumbler over ice.
Makes 200 ml (7 fl oz)

Nutritional values

- Kcals 180
- Vitamin A 70,654 iu
- Vitamin C 105 mg
- Selenium 5 mcg
- Zinc 0.95 mg

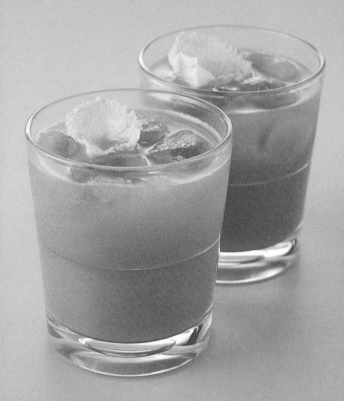

CONSTIPATION. A sluggish digestive system, caused by poor diet and lack of digestive enzymes, can cause constipation, an uncomfortable affliction which may lead to blockage and distension of the bowel. A combination of fruit and vegetables high in fibre and cleansing properties will help to exercise and stimulate the abdomen and improve digestion. This juice really could be called a lethal weapon – a dose of three potent laxatives that will get you back on line.

way to go

250 g (8 oz) pear
25 g (1 oz) pitted prunes
125 g (4 oz) spinach

Juice all the ingredients and serve in a glass over ice cubes. Decorate with pear slices, if liked.
Makes 200 ml (7 fl oz)

Nutritional values

- Kcals 302
- Vitamin A 8,946 iu
- Vitamin C 80 mg
- Potassium 1,311 mg

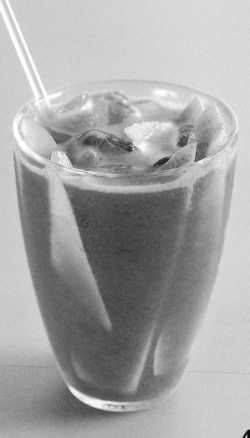

49

DIARRHOEA. Whether you're suffering from food poisoning, stress, travel sickness or jet-lag, diarrhoea will dehydrate your system. This means you must ensure that your body gets plenty of liquids to replace the nutrients lost. Blueberries contain anthocyanosides, which are lethal to the bacteria that can cause diarrhoea.

belly berry

250 g (8 oz) apple
125 g (4 oz) blueberries,
fresh or frozen

Juice the apple, then whizz in a blender with the blueberries. Serve in a tumbler.
Makes 150 ml (¼ pint)

Nutritional values

- Kcals 210
- Vitamin A 8.946 iu
- Vitamin C 20 mg
- Magnesium 18.5 mg

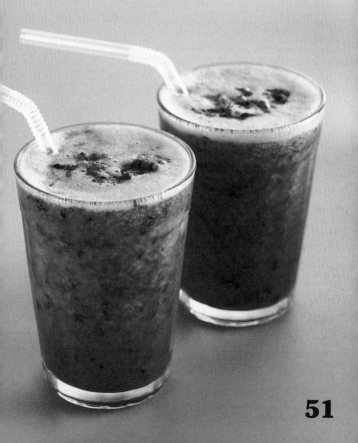

51

ARTHRITIS. The most common form of arthritis, whereby the smooth layer of cartilage that covers and cushions the ends of the bones gradually breaks down, mainly affects elderly people. The swollen and inflamed joints that result are an extremely painful condition. There are many foods that can ease the discomfort of this complaint including cabbage, citrus fruits, berries and fruits high in vitamin C. The salicylic acid in grapefruit works to break down uric acid deposits and the carrot and spinach help to rebuild and regenerate cartilage and joints.

twister

125 g (4 oz) pink
  grapefruit
125 g (4 oz) carrot
125 g (4 oz) spinach

Peel the grapefruit, keeping as much of the pith as possible. Juice all the ingredients and serve in a tumbler. Decorate with slices of grapefruit, if liked.
Makes 200 ml (7 fl oz)

Nutritional values

- Kcals 185
- Vitamin A 43,864 iu
- Vitamin C 167 mg
- Cysteine 43 mg

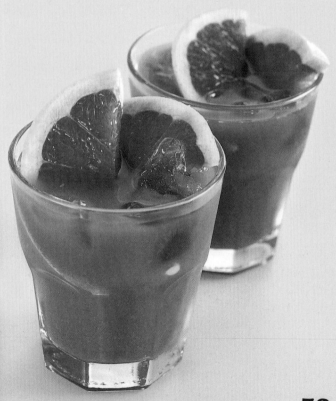

53

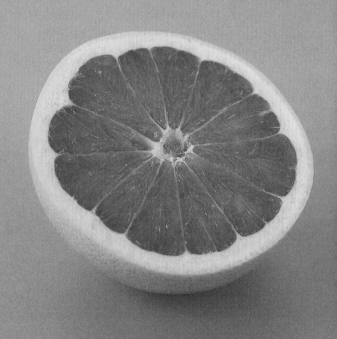

fitness

OSTEOPOROSIS. This is a debilitating disease, and, although it primarily affects women who have gone through the menopause, it is imperative that even women in their twenties supplement their eating plan with bone-strengthening foods. Turnip-top leaves contain more calcium than milk. Broccoli is also ideal, as it also contains calcium and folic acid. Dandelion leaves are excellent sources of magnesium, which helps the body utilize the calcium for healthy bones and teeth.

sticks and stones

125 g (4 oz) turnip,
  including the tops
125 g (4 oz) carrot
125 g (4 oz) broccoli
handful of dandelion
  leaves
175 g (6 oz) apple

Scrub the turnip and carrot. Juice all the ingredients and whizz in a blender with a couple of ice cubes. Serve in a tall glass decorated with dandelion leaves, if liked.
Makes 200 ml (7 fl oz)

Nutritional values

- Kcals 196
- Vitamin A 50,391 iu
- Vitamin C 223 mg
- Magnesium 108 mg
- Calcium 398 mg
- Folic acid 210 mcg

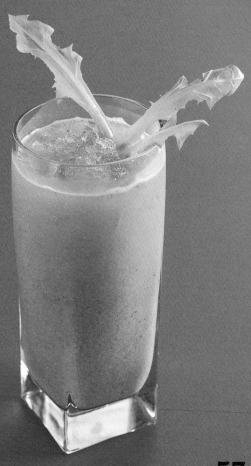

57

EYESIGHT. Remember when your mother nagged you to eat your carrots, so that you could see in the dark? Well, she was right, as carrots contain high levels of beta-carotene and vitamin E, which are necessary for maintaining healthy eyes. Endive is helpful in preventing cataracts. This combination of vegetables provides a high vitamin A content that nourishes the optic nerve.

vision
impeccable

175 g (6 oz) carrot
125 g (4 oz) endive
125 g (4 oz) celery

Juice the carrot, endive and celery. Whizz in a blender with a couple of ice cubes and serve decorated with lemon slices and some chopped parsley, if liked.
Makes 200 ml (7 fl oz)

Nutritional values

- Kcals 128
- Vitamin A 53,687 iu
- Vitamin C 33 mg
- Potassium 1,499 mg

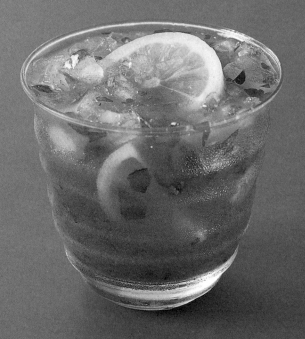

59

PREGNANCY CARE. Eating (or juicing) for two may seem overwhelming when you are first pregnant, but you do not need to double your intake of nutrients and vitamins although it is recommended that you increase several of them. Nutritionists advise that, for most women, an additional 200 calories per day is all that's required therefore juicing is a great way to increase your intake of nutrients whilst controlling your calorie count. More importantly, though, ensure that you eat (or juice) foods high in folic acid, to reduce the possibility of spina bifida. This juice is rich in folic acid and vitamin A, which are essential for foetal development and guard against pre-eclampsia.

earth mother

125 g (4 oz) carrot
125 g (4 oz) lettuce
125 g (4 oz) parsnip
125 g (4 oz) cantaloupe
   melon

Juice the carrot, lettuce and parsnip with the flesh of the melon. Serve in a tall glass with wedges of melon, if liked.
Makes 200 ml (7 fl oz)

Nutritional values

• Kcals 204
• Vitamin A 42,136 iu
• Vitamin C 115 mg
• Folic acid 93.75 mcg
• Fat 2.1 g

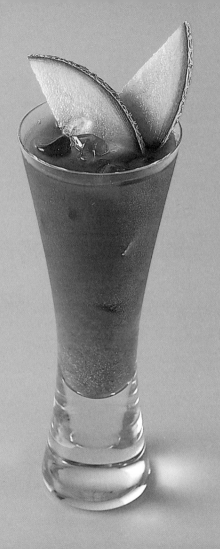

61

MUSCLE DAMAGE. Athletes often suffer muscle damage during training and, even with precautions, often seem to attract bangs, knocks and other injuries. Ensuring that there is enough vitamin C in your diet helps protect against muscle damage, and leads to a reduction in muscle soreness and improved general healing. Vitamin C may also help to increase oxygen uptake and aerobic energy production. Weight for weight, kiwi fruits contain more vitamin C than oranges.

healing hand

2 ripe pears
3 kiwi fruits
½ lime

Wash the pears, peel the kiwi fruits and scrub the lime. Slice the fruit into even-sized pieces then juice. Pour into a glass, add a couple of ice cubes and decorate with slices of kiwi fruit, if liked.
Makes 300 ml (½ pint)

Nutritional values

- Kcals 210
- Protein 3 g
- Vitamin C 130 mg
- Calcium 80 mg
- Iron 1.3 mg

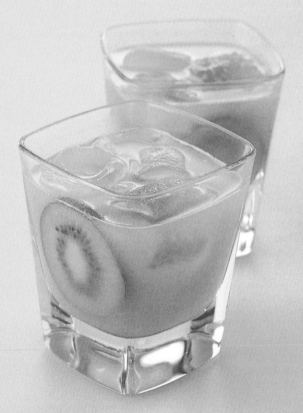

63

index

acknowledgements

The publisher would like to thank The Juicer Company
for the loan of The Champion juicer and the Orange X
citrus juicer (featured on pages 12 and 13).

Executive Editor Nicola Hill
Editor Rachel Lawrence
Executive Art Editor Geoff Fennell
Designer Sue Michniewicz
Senior Production Controller Jo Sim
Photographer Stephen Conroy
Home Economist David Morgan
Stylist Angela Swaffield
All photographs © Octopus
Publishing Group Ltd